T0214291

lower than an arbitrary cutoff, the null hypothesis th. the values of that parameter in the two populations alternative hypothesis (i.e., the two values are diffe. ╌╌╌╌ ₁୨୨ͻ). Note that the alternative hypothesis can also be more specific about the difference between the two values of the parameters (in terms of the direction of the difference). Nevertheless, to obtain valid and useful results, it is necessary that they derive from an appropriately designed investigation with an adequate statistical power.

Statistical power is commonly defined as "a test's ability to detect a difference when it actually exists" (Wittes 2002). To analyze the statistical power of a study, the following parameters must be considered (Jekel 1996):

- Level of significance α (probability of type I error, that is the probability to reject the null hypothesis when is true)
- Statistical power
- Difference to detect (effect size)
- Variance of the main measure
- Sample size.

These five parameters are not independent: Indeed, if you know four of them, the fifth can be easily calculated.

Based on this premise, the objective of power analysis is usually to calculate the needed sample size knowing the values of the other parameters. The importance of a priori sample size calculation is often underrated, or even ignored, since it is rarely executed, despite being of critical importance for the effective usefulness of a study's results (Pandis et al. 2011). Unfortunately, in the clinical setting sample size is often conditioned or even limited by the number of available or recruitable subjects, thus exposing to several risks when interpreting results of the study.

For example, in case of a randomized clinical trial, if sample size (N) is small, the study could not have enough statistical power to detect real differences between two treatment modalities and, therefore, a "negative result" (i.e., absence of differences) should not be useful. So, negative results have their usefulness only if N is big enough to detect real differences. On the contrary, if N is too big, it could be detected a difference having no clinical importance. This last problem may affect the interpretation of findings from meta-analyses performed by meshing results of many investigations, where the large sample size may condition the detection of statistically, but not clinically, significant differences. Considering that, a priori sample size calculation is strongly recommended, as its estimation could reveal, for example, that the number of subjects necessary to detect a determined statistical significance is so high that the study is not practicable, or it is lower than expected, consenting to avoid useless efforts.

Formulae for sample size calculation are different for each type of study, but all derive from the following base equation (Machin et al. 1997):

N (for each group) $= (Z_\alpha + Z_\beta)^2 \times 2 \times S^2/D^2$

where N = sample size per group; $Z_\alpha = \alpha$-quantile of a standard normal distribution; $Z_\beta = \beta$-quantile of a standard normal distribution, where β is the type II error (i.e., the probability to not reject a null hypothesis when is not true); $S^2 =$ variance; D = difference to detect.

Before suggesting how to apply sample size calculation formulae to studies on TMD, it is necessary to review some essential terms, concepts and steps on which those formulae are based.

1.3.1   The Choice of an Evaluation Measure

The first step for sample size calculation is to decide which is the main variable among those investigated for differences between two populations or two treatment modalities. The importance of the main variable has not to be underrated. Indeed, many studies deal with more than one outcome measure, whether in case of assessment measures to evaluate efficacy of two treatment modalities or in case of the prevalence of more than one feature in different populations. In those cases, the most clinically meaningful or epidemiologically relevant variable must be considered the main evaluation measure.

1.3.2   Alpha Error (Type I Error)

It is defined as the risk to have a false-positive result, that is to have a statistically significant difference when it does not exist (Pocock et al. 1987). Alpha is conventionally set at 0.05, therefore accepting a 5 % probability to fall into a false-positive error. A small alpha value means that its corresponding Z value (Z_α) is big (in absolute value). For example, an alpha value of 0.05 corresponds to a Z_α value of ± 1.64. In case of an alpha value reduced to 0.01 (1 % risk of a false-positive result), the corresponding Z_α should be ± 2.33. Therefore, it is intuitive that the lower the risk to have a false-positive result, the higher the sample size, since in the base equation Z_α is numerator.

1.3.3   Beta Error (Type II Error)

It is defined as the risk to have a false-negative result, that is to not detect a significant difference when it actually exists (Pocock et al. 1987). This type of error could happen when a clinically important difference is not statistically significant due to the small sample size. Therefore, a study with a high beta error has a low sensitivity to detect a difference. Sensitivity is usually expressed in terms of "statistical power," in the sense that statistical power + beta error = 1.00. So, statistical power is 1−beta error. Statistical power is defined as the ability of a study to detect a real difference. It is often conventionally set at 80 % (beta error = 0.20), being only rarely increased up to 90 % or 95 %. The reasons to accept such a low statistical power, with a 20 % risk to lose a true result, have not a scientific basis, and they are more pragmatic than logical. A beta value of 0.20 means the corresponding Z_β is 0.84.

1.3.4 Variance of the Main Outcome Measure

The variance of an observed data set is defined as the sum of quadratic standard deviations, divided for the number of observations minus 1 (Freiman et al. 1978). Therefore, a high variance causes high risks of uncertainty when estimating the mean value of a data set. Such risks, as it is intuitive, have to be reduced and compensated by increasing the sample size, since the variance is numerator in the base equation.

1.3.5 Difference to Detect

The last parameter to set for sample size calculation is the difference a researcher is willing to detect between the groups. This difference must have clinical importance and, with the exception of some existing conventions, must derive from the experience and the opinion of researchers. Another intuitive aspect is that the smaller the difference we want to detect, the bigger the sample size necessary to detect it. For example, if a drug A can decrease arterial blood pressure 1 mmHg more than a drug B, such difference could be statistically significant only in a large-sized sample. Such a study should be surely expensive in terms of money and efforts, and should be a nonsense, unless such a small difference is clinically important or the use of the drug A has strong advantages on the drug B (for example, a lower cost or an easier availability).

1.4 Sample Size Calculation for Studies on TMD

Some meta-analyses evidenced that a priori sample size calculation is an often ignored step in the medical literature (Moher et al. 1994). For example, a review on about 300 randomized clinical trials (RCT) with negative results (i.e., no differences between the evaluated treatment modalities have been detected) evidenced that only 7% of those studies had a statistical power of at least 80% to detect a 25% difference in efficacy, and 31% were capable to detect a 50% difference (Freiman et al. 1978). That means the negative results of most of those studies could have been a consequence of the poor statistical power and the small sample size. Despite according to some authors the so-called beta-error problem has been overrated, such review paper has been extensively cited in the medical literature as an example of how flaws in the internal validity of a study's findings can be detected. The number of works with an appropriate statistical power was only slightly increased in the years which followed such the publication (for example, in a sample of RCT with negative results published in 1990, only 16% had enough power to detect a 25% difference and 36% to evidence a 50% difference) (Moher et al. 1994).

Such observations, even though there is no report on this issue, are probably applicable also to the studies on TMD for a number of reasons, among which the relative youth of those conditions and also the difficulties to design high-quality studies in this specific field of research.

When designing studies on TMD, the first step to calculate sample size is the choice of an appropriate assessment measure. This is not a problem in case of observational or descriptive studies (e.g., prevalence of an accompanying pathology or condition in a population of TMD subjects versus prevalence in a control group; percentage of TMD subjects with a particular occlusal feature versus percentage of subjects at a population level; mean scores of a population of TMD subjects in a test or a questionnaire versus mean scores of a group of healthy subjects, etc.), but it could represent an error source, if not correctly identified, in case of clinical trials evaluating the treatment efficacy of two different therapeutic approaches. Indeed, a valid outcome measure must accurately represent the phenomena being studied and must be capable of reflecting real changes in patient's condition.

1.4.1 Longitudinal Studies

In case of clinical trials, the peculiar nature of pain conditions, such as TMD, makes impossible to compare the treatment efficacy of two therapeutic modalities in term of success versus failure due to the fluctuation of symptoms and the complexity of pain experience. A number of assessment measures has been proposed for TMD patients, such as recording of joint sounds, patterns of jaw movement, and electromyographic activity of the masticatory muscles. Unfortunately, because of their low sensitivity and specificity, their use as an outcome variable to evaluate treatment efficacy cannot be supported (Lund et al. 1995; Manfredini et al. 2012a; Manfredini et al. 2013a).

Some authors proposed a method to quantify the smallest clinically detectable difference of mouth opening and mandibular functioning, suggesting that such parameter should be the starting point to evaluate the validity and the clinical significance of post-treatment changes (Kropmans et al. 1999). Others proposed to rely on the patient's subjective feeling of pain relief to evaluate treatment efficacy, but this measure is clearly exposed to subject bias, since at the end of treatment patients often tend to overrate their pre-treatment pain (Feine et al. 1989).

Because of the poor reliability of the above-described techniques, the best outcome measure for clinical trials on TMD patients still remains the Visual Analogue Scale (VAS) (Price et al. 1983). The VAS scale is a broadly employed, simple, rapid, and valid method to assess pain, both in clinical than in experimental conditions. VAS, mostly in the form with anchor points to make easier the patient's visualization of pain, gives a sensitive and accurate description of pain (Duncan et al. 1989).

The main objections against the systematic introduction of VAS as the main outcome variable for TMD treatments could be that pain is not a common characteristic for all conditions grouped under the term "TMD" and that it is not suitable to define the complex multifaceted pain experience. Anyhow, it can be viewed as the most immediate outcome measure to define the needed sample size because of its simplicity and its diffusion around the medical literature, thus making easy to find some existing data on different topics.

Once VAS has been chosen as the main outcome variable, it is necessary to select an appropriate difference to be sought. As a rule of thumb, it must be borne in mind that a statistically significant difference is not necessarily clinically significant, so that the number of subjects included in the study should be adequate but not excessive, in order to reveal the presence or the absence of differences having both a clinical and statistical significance.

An important work by Ekblom and Hansson underlined that a 15 % decrease in VAS ratings was interpreted by subjects as being insignificant (Ekblom and Hansson 1988). On the opposite hand, it is rare, if not impossible, to find large differences (e.g., 80 % or more) between two treatment modalities. This is mostly true in case of TMD for which the percentage of success of the various therapeutic approaches is high (Manfredini 2010). On that purpose, Clark et al. showed that the fluctuant nature of the symptoms and the high rate of spontaneous remission characterizing myofascial pain lead to a rate of improvement of about 26 % in non-treated patients (Clark et al. 1988). According to Dao et al., a clinically significant improvement is a 40 % decrease in VAS ratings (Dao et al. 1994). Such value, in our opinion, should be considered the standard of reference for planning the sample size for a clinical trial on TMD patients.

An example of a randomized clinical trial with negative results is a work comparing treatment effectiveness of traditional acupuncture and sham acupuncture, viz., application of needles in non-conventional areas, on patients affected by myofascial pain (Goddard et al. 2002). The authors concluded that no significant outcome differences exist between traditional and sham acupuncture, since both caused a decrease in VAS ratings. Actually, data analysis revealed that VAS ratings decrease was higher in patients treated with traditional acupuncture than in those treated with sham acupuncture. Such difference was about 13 points in VAS ratings. It was not significant due to the small sample size (18 subjects in total), but it actually represented about 20 % of the mean pre-treatment VAS score. Power analysis revealed that the authors should have needed 85 subjects per group to detect a 25 % difference in treatment effectiveness between the groups, and 33 subjects per group to detect a 40 % difference. Therefore, the study did not have enough statistical power to detect a real difference, if it had existed.

1.4.2 Cross-Sectional Studies

In case of non-longitudinal studies, the first thing to consider is the nature of the main variable. In most cases, it is either continuous, viz., expressed as a numeric value, or dichotomic, viz., expressed as presence/absence.

An example of a cross-sectional study with a numeric main variable is the comparison of mean scores in a test or a questionnaire between a population of TMD patients and a group of TMD-free subjects. This kind of investigations employ questionnaires designed, for example, to rate different aspects related with the psychosocial sphere, such as the quality of life (e.g., MPI), anxiety (e.g., STAI) or depressive disorders (e.g., BDI), or broader spectra of psychopathology. In these investigations, information on the estimated variance must derive from analogue studies in the literature or from preliminary data drawn from pilot studies, while the difference to detect must be suggested by clinical considerations or by psychometric properties of the adopted measures. The formula to calculate sample size is the same described for clinical trials.

An example of study with a dichotomic main variable is an investigation which compares the prevalence of bruxism in the general population and that in a sample of TMD subjects. In this case, both the variance and the difference to detect are expressed in terms of percentage, or even better proportions, of bruxers. Calculating the variance is easy, being approximately the product of mean proportion of bruxers (mean percentage of bruxers subjects between the TMD group and the general population) and its complement to 1.

In this case, the equation to calculate sample size is the following:

N (for each group) $=(Z_\alpha+Z_\beta)^2\times 2\times P(1-P)/D^2$,

where N, D, Z_α, and Z_β maintain their significance, and $P(1-P)$ is the variance.

For example, data from the literature suggest that self-report diagnosed bruxism has a prevalence of about 20% at population level (Manfredini et al. 2013b) and it is about twice as prevalent in TMD patients (Manfredini et al. 2012b). In a study on two samples of the same dimension, mean prevalence should be 30% (proportion 0.3) and the estimated variance should be $0.3\times 0.7=0.21$. The difference between the groups should be 20% (0.2). If we would consider such difference clinically significant, to statistically detect it, we should need

$N=(1.96+0.84)^2\times 2\times(0.3\times 0.7)/(0.2)^2=82.25$ subjects per group.

Another study in which the same formula for sample size calculation should be adopted is an investigation on the association between a particular occlusal feature and TMD. Pullinger and Seligman suggested that a risk factor, in their case represented by a number of occlusal variables, has to reach at least a 2:1 odds ratio for disease to be considered potentially clinically relevant. The same authors observed also that such threshold is not always related with actual statistical significance, since the latter can be detected even for lower odds ratios (Pullinger and Seligman 2000). Given those considerations, if a particular occlusal feature has a prevalence of about 15% at population level, a 2:1 relative risk for TMD will be achieved for a prevalence of 30% in a sample of TMD patients. To detect this difference we should need

$N=(1.96+0.84)^2\times 2\times(0.225\times 0.775)/(0.15)^2=118.22$ subjects per group.

1.5   Different Types of Clinically Oriented Researches

Sample size calculation is a basic step in a study design. Nevertheless, as shown by several works in the literature, it is often ignored. Thus, even without dealing with all the possible casuistry of studies on TMD, the above rules may be useful to calculate the sample size necessary for studies on those conditions as well as to sensitize researchers with regard to this issue.

A correct design is essential for the effective usefulness of results, both in longitudinal and in cross-sectional investigations. Notwithstanding that, choosing the appropriate sample size is not the only mandatory pre-requisite for performing a good research.

In the field of TMD and orofacial pain, an important amount of research is based on the so-called basic experiments testing, for example, motor reflexes, reaction to experimental pain, and physiological responses to different stimuli. Notwithstanding that, a direct transfer of such knowledge to the clinical setting is often limited in the short-time span after the publication of basic research studies. On the contrary, clinically oriented researches have a much stronger influence on the daily practitioner's perspectives, and they represent a good source for providing easy-to-understand examples on the different statistical designs that can be adopted to answer a clinical research question. Some very interesting publications exist to provide readers with some suggestions for designing a patient-oriented research that can enhance the manuscript readability and data comprehension by the clinical community (Dodson 2007).

Once the need for performing a patient-oriented research has been established, several different types of study designs can be adopted depending on the aims to pursue. Investigations in the field of TMD can be directed to get deeper into the etiology or epidemiology of the disease as well as the diagnostic and therapeutic concepts. Also, systematic literature reviews cannot be underestimated as a source of useful evidence-based information for clinical and research purposes.

Studies on the epidemiological features of TMD and orofacial pain patients should report accurately as many data as available on both axis I, viz., physical, and axis II, viz., psychosocial, diagnoses, according to the currently accepted view that multidimensional assessment of pain features is of paramount importance in the clinical setting. Also, the natural course of disease should be assessed and reported according to structured reporting guidelines (e.g., Strenghtening the Reporting of Observational Studies in Epidemiology (STROBE)) (Von Elm et al. 2007), in order to provide data for comparison of treatment effects. At the etiological level, most investigations explored putative risk factors for disease. To do that, several study designs can be adopted, ranging from "simple" single variable to "complex" multiple variable analyses, with the latter being much more suitable to support "strong" conclusions.

Most part of the TMD and orofacial pain literature focused on the diagnostic and therapeutic issues, with several possible strategies to design, perform, and report investigations on various arguments. The main reasoning underlying any study on TMD diagnosis is that a reliable diagnostic marker should be established and, if pain levels are assumed as such, any clinical, instrumental, or laboratory examinations must be assessed for the accuracy to distinguish between subjects with and without pain. Treatment studies can be either case series or clinical trials, with the latter allowing several interesting study designs.

Finally, it must be borne in mind that the highest rank in the hierarchy of scientific evidence is occupied by high-quality literature review summarizing all the available peer-reviewed studies on a particular topic by performing either qualitative or structurally reported assessments.

Based on these premises, examples of study designs will be provided in the remaining sections of the book.

References

Bland M. An introduction to medical statistics. 2nd ed. Oxford: Oxford Medical Publications; 1995.

Clark GT, Lanham F, Flack VF. Treatment outcome results for consecutive TMJ clinic patients. J Craniomandib Disord. 1988;2:87–95.

Dao TTT, Lavigne GJ, Feine JS, Tanguay R, Lund JP. Power and sample size calculations for clinical trials of myofascial pain of jaw muscles. J Dent Res. 1991;70:118–22.

De Boever JA, Nilner M, Orthlieb JD, Steenks MH. Recommendations by the EACD for examination, diagnosis, and management of patients with temporomandibular disorders and orofacial pain by the general dental practitioner. J Orofac Pain. 2008;22:268–78.

De Laat A, Stappaers K, Papy S. Counseling and physical therapy as treatment for myofascial pain of the masticatory system. J Orofac Pain. 2003; 17:42–9.

De Leeuw R. Internal derangements of the temporomandibular joint. Oral Maxillofac Surg Clin North Am. 2008a;20:159–68.

De Leeuw R. The American academy of orofacial pain. Orofacial pain: guidelines for assessment, diagnosis, and management. Chicago: Quintessence Publishing; 2008b.

Dionne RA. Pharmacologic treatment of acute and chronic orofacial pain. Oral Maxillofac Surg Clin North Am. 2000;12:309–20.

Dodson TB. A guide for preparing a patient-oriented research manuscript. Oral Surg Oral Med Oral Pathol Oral Radiol Endod. 2007;104:307–15.

Dolwick MF, Dimitroulis G. Is there a role for temporomandibular joint surgery? Brit J Oral Maxillofac Surg. 1994;32:307–13.

Duncan GH, Bushnell MC, Lavigne GJ. Comparison of verbal and visual analogue scales for measuring the intensity and unpleasantness of experimental pain. Pain. 1989;37:295–303.

Dworkin SF, Leresche L. Research diagnostic criteria for temporomandibular disorders: review, criteria, examinations and specifications, critique. J Craniomandib Disord. 1992;6:301–55.

Ekblom A, Hansson P. Pain intensity measurements in patients with acute pain receiving afferent stimulation. J Neurol Neurosurg Psychiatry. 1988;51:481–6.

Feine JS, Dao TTT, Lavigne GJ, Lund JP. Is treatment success due to faulty memory of chronic pain? J Dent Res. 1989; 68:1018 (abstract).

Freiman JA, Chalmers TC, Smith H, Kuebler RR. The importance of beta, the type II error, and sample size in the design and interpretation of the randomized controlled trial: survey of 71 "negative" trials. N Engl J Med. 1978;299:690–4.

Gatchel RJ, Stowell AW, Wildenstein L, Riggs R, Ellis E. Efficacy of an early intervention for patients with acute TMD-related pain: a one-year outcome study. J Am Dent Assoc. 2006;137:339–47.

Gavish A, Winocur E, Astandzelov-Nachmias T, Gazit E. Effect of controlled masticatory exercise on pain and muscle performance in myofascial pain patients: a pilot study. Cranio. 2006;24:184–90.

Goddard G, Karibe H, McNeill C, Villafuerte E. Acupuncture and sham acupuncture reduce muscle pain in myofascial pain patients. J Orofac Pain. 2002;16:71–6.

Greene C. Concepts of TMD etiology: effects on diagnosis and treatment. In: Laskin DM, Greene CS, Hylander WL, editors. TMDs: an evidence-based approach to diagnosis and treatment. Chicago: Quintessence Publishing; 2006a. p. 219–28.

Greene CS. Science transfer in orofacial pain. In: Lund JP, Lavigne GJ, Dubner R, Sessle BJ, editors. Orofacial pain: from basic science to clinical management. Chicago: Quintessence Publishing; 2006b. p. 281–86.

Guarda-Nardini L, Stifano M, Brombin C, Salmaso L, Manfredini D. A one-year case series of arthrocentesis with hyaluronic acid injections for temporomandibular joint osteoarthritis. Oral Surg Oral Med Oral Pathol Oral Radiol Endod. 2007;103:e14–22.

Guarda-Nardini L, Manfredini D, Ferronato G. Temporomandibular joint total replacement prosthesis: current knowledge and considerations for the future. Int J Oral Maxillofac Surg. 2008;37:103–10.

Jekel J. Epidemiology, biostatistics and preventive medicine. Philadelphia: W.B. Saunders Company; 1996.

Klasser GD, Greene CS. Oral appliances in the management of temporomandibular disorders. Oral Surg Oral Med Oral Pathol Oral Radiol Endod. 2009a;107:212–23.

Klasser GD, Greene CS. The changing field of temporomandibular disorders: what dentists need to know. J Can Dent Assoc. 2009b;75:49–53.

Koh H, Robinson PG. Occlusal adjustment for treating and preventing temporomandibular joint disorders. Cochrane Database Syst Rev. 2003;(1):CD003812.

Kropmans TJB, Stegenga B, Dijkstra PU, Van Veen A. The smallest detectable difference of mandibular function impairment in patients with a painfully restricted temporomandibular joint. J Dent Res. 1999;78:1445–9.

Laskin DM. Etiology of the pain-dysfunction syndrome. J Am Dent Assoc. 1969;79:147–53.

Lund JP, Widmer CG, Feine JS. Validity of diagnostic and monitoring tests used for temporomandibular disorders. J Dent Res. 1995;74:1133–43.

Machin D, Campbell MJ, Fayers PM, Pinol APY. Sample size tables for clinical studies. 2nd ed. Oxford: Blackwell Science; 1997.

Magnusson T, Egermark I, Carlsson GE. A prospective investigation over two decades on signs and symptoms of temporomandibular disorders and associated variables. A final summary. Acta Odontol Scand. 2005;63:99–109.

Manfredini D. Fundamentals of TMD management. In: Manfredini D, editor. Current concepts on temporomandibular disorders. Berlin: Quintessence Publishing; 2010a. p. 305–18.

Manfredini D. Integration of research into the clinical practice. In: Manfredini D, editor. Current concepts on temporomandibular disorders. Berlin: Quintessence Publishing; 2010b. p. 459–68.

Manfredini D, Tognini F, Biondi K, Bosco M. Sample size calculation for studies on temporomandibular disorders. Minerva Stomatol. 2003;52:309–19.

Manfredini D, Chiappe G, Bosco M. Research diagnostic criteria for temporomandibular disorders (RDC/TMD) axis I diagnosis in an italian patients population. J Oral Rehabil. 2006;33:551–8.

Manfredini D, Piccotti F, Ferronato G, Guarda-Nardini L. Age peaks of different RDC/TMD diagnoses in a patient population. J Dent. 2010;38:392–9.

Manfredini D, Castroflorio T, Perinetti G, Guarda-Nardini L. Dental occlusion, body posture, and temporomandibular disorders: where we are now and where we are heading for. J Oral Rehabil. 2012a;39:463–71.

Manfredini D, Winocur E, Guarda-Nardini L, Lobbezoo F. Self-reported bruxism and temporomandibular disorders: findings from two specialised centers. J Oral Rehabil. 2012b;39:319–25.

Manfredini D, Favero L, Michieli M, Salmaso L, Cocilovo F, Guarda-Nardini L. Assessment of jaw kinesiography to monitor temporomandibular disorders: correlation of treatment-related kinesiographic and pain changes in patients undergoing TMJ injections. J Am Dent Assoc. 2013a;144:397–405.

Manfredini D, Winocur E, Guarda-Nardini L, Paesani D, Lobbezoo F. Epidemiology of bruxism in adults: a systematic review of literature. J Orofac Pain. 2013b;27:99–110.

Moher D, Dulberg C, Wells G. Statistical power, sample size, and their reporting in randomized controlled trials. JAMA. 1994;272:122–4.

Nitzan DW, Dolwick MF, Martinez GA. Temporomandibular joint arthrocentesis: a simplified treatment for severe, limited mouth opening. J Oral Maxillofac Surg. 1991;49:1163–7.

Okeson JP. The classification of orofacial pains. Oral Maxillofac Surg Clin N Am. 2008;20:133–44.

Pandis N, Polychronopoulou A, Eliades T. Sample size estimation: an overview with applications to orthodontic clinical trial designs. Am J Orthod Dentofacial Orthop. 2011;140:141–6.

Pocock SJ, Hughes MD, Lee RJ. Statistical problems in the reporting of clinical trials: a survey of three medical journals. N Engl J Med. 1987;317:426–32.

Price DD, McGrath PA, Rafii A, Buckingham B. The validation of Visual Analogue Scales as ratio scale measures for chronic and experimental pain. Pain. 1983;17:45–56.

Pullinger A, Seligman D. Quantification and validation of predictive values of occlusal variables in temporomandibular disorders using a multifactorial analysis. J Prosthet Dent. 2000;83:66–75.

Rollmann GB, Gillespie JM. The role of psychosocial factors in temporomandibular disorders. Curr Rev Pain. 2000;4:71–81.

Schiffmann E, Fricton JR, Harley D, Shapiro BL. The prevalence and treatment needs of subjects with temporomandibular disorders. J Am Dent Assoc. 1990;120:295–304.

Schiffman E, Ohrbach R, Truelove E, Look J, Anderson G, Goulet JP, List T, Svensson P, Gonzalez Y, Lobbezoo F, Michelotti A, Brooks SL, Ceusters W, Drangsholt M, Ettlin D, Gaul C, Goldberg LJ, Haythornthwaite JA, Hollender L, Jensen R, John MT, De Laat A, de Leeuw R, Maixner W, van der Meulen M, Murray GM, Nixdorf DR, Palla S, Petersson A, Pionchon P, Smith B, Visscher CM, Zakrzewska J, Dworkin SF. Diagnostic criteria for temporomandibular disorders (DC/TMD) for clinical and research applications: recommendations of the international RDC/TMD consortium network* and orofacial pain special interest group†. J Oral Facial Pain Headache. 2014;28:6–27.

Stohler C, Zarb G. On the management of temporomandibular disorders: a plea for low-tech, high-prudence therapeutic approach. J Orofac Pain. 1999;13:255–61.

Turp JC, Schindler HJ. Occlusal therapy of temporomandibular pain. In: Manfredini D, editor. Current concepts on temporomandibular disorders. Berlin: Quintessence Publishing; 2010. p. 359–82.

Turp JC, Greene CS, Strub JR. Dental occlusion: a critical reflection on past, present and future concepts. J Oral Rehabil. 2008;35:446–53.

Von Elm E, Altman DG, Egger M, Pocock SJ, Gotzsche PC, Vandenbroucke JP. The strengthening the reporting of observational studies in epidemiology (STROBE) statement: guidelines for reporting observational studies. Ann Intern Med. 2007;147:573–7.

Wittes J. Sample size calculations for randomised controlled trials. Epidemiol Rev. 2002;24:39–53.

Chapter 2
Etiology and Epidemiology

Daniele Manfredini and Luca Guarda-Nardini

In the present chapter, which is dedicated to the provision of examples of the different strategies to investigate for the role of etiological/risk factors and to report data for epidemiological purposes, the main focus is put on two aspects that represent the fil rouge of the various investigations here described. The first issue is related with the epidemiology of the temporomandibular disorders (TMDs), the description of which must forcedly take into account for the psychosocial features of the disease, as suggested by the biopsychosocial model of orofacial pain. The need to describe and report as many details as possible on the so-called axis II impairment is well-exampled in the large-sample study commented in the section on how to report epidemiology data. The second issue, which is strictly related to the other, is related with the shift from past beliefs of an importance of dental occlusion in the etiology and bruxism to the current concepts providing that a triangle of factors, viz., bruxism, pain, and psychosocial factors, may explain most part of the pathogenesis of TMDs. Three example investigations are provided on the topic of the etiology of bruxism and TMDs, all authored by two of this book's editors. The materials and methods as well as the results sections will be edited with respect to the original publication, especially by providing specific comments on the different clinical and statistical strategies underlying the study rationale. Taken together, the information contained in this chapter succeeds to reach the twofold aim of providing suggestions for clinical purposes (i.e., presentation of the current concepts on TMD epidemiology and etiology) as well as for statistical uses (i.e., discussion of the various models that need to be adopted for some different research situations and/or to test different hypotheses).

D. Manfredini (✉) · L. Guarda-Nardini
University of Padova, Padova, Italy
e-mail: daniele.manfredini@tin.it

L. Guarda-Nardini
e-mail: luca.guarda@unipd.it

L. Salmaso et al., *Statistical Approaches to Orofacial Pain and Temporomandibular Disorders Research,* SpringerBriefs in Statistics, DOI 10.1007/978-1-4939-0876-9_2, © The Author(s) 2014

2.1   The Need to Get Deeper Into Etiology and Define Epidemiology

In an ideal condition, a correct diagnosis and an effective treatment for a disease should be based on the knowledge about the etiology and pathophysiology of the disease. A known pathophysiology provides the identification of an etiologic agent and the description of the pathogenetic mechanism leading to the onset of the disease and to its natural course. A thorough knowledge of all these aspects is of basic importance to allow a sensible diagnosis and treatment planning.

In the case of TMDs, most part of the past century was dominated by the so-called occlusal etiology paradigm, which met consensus by the majority of clinicians and researchers. In accordance with such an occlusal paradigm, the diagnosis was focused on the assessment of dental occlusion and the treatment was based on irreversible changes of dental occlusion itself. Successively, in the last decades of the past century, several authors raised concerns about the conceptual validity of the occlusal etiology theory and, conversely, an increasing number of papers showed that patients with pain in the facial area shared many characteristics with patients affected by other chronic pain diseases in terms of psychological distress, social impairment, and reduced quality of life. These observations, along with the evolution of concepts about pain perception and modulation, put the basis for the first multidimensional pain model for TMD patients (Rollmann and Gillespie 2000; Suvinen et al. 2005).

The next step provided that the biological disorder was seen within the frame of illness experience (i.e., reactions to the physical disorders), thus leading to the biopsychosocial model for TMD and its derived terminology and classification (Dworkin and Leresche 1992). The biopsychosocial model for TMD, which is still considered the best-fitting model for TMD assessment, has to be taken into full account when reporting findings of any kind of investigations in the field of TMD and orofacial pain.

Based on these premises, examples of how to report data on TMD epidemiology will be provided in the remaining sections of this chapter as well as examples of different study design to get deeper into the etiology of TMD to add data to the multifactorial model of TMD and orofacial pain.

2.2   How to Report Data on Epidemiology

Clinicians and researchers approaching to medical data gathering/presenting and to manuscript writing must start with a clear definition of their objectives. The following is an example introduction for an epidemiology-based research, featuring two main characteristics:

1. A logical presentation of the study aims and rationale, viz., the need to get deeper into the epidemiology of this specific disease, along with hints to the currently available literature
2. A brief description of the instrument(s) used to perform the investigation, to be presented in greater detail later in the successive sections.

2.2.1 Statement of the Problem

As in all other fields of pain medicine, there is a strong need to define treatment-seeking populations in terms of their different patterns of signs and symptoms distribution, viz., the relative percentage of patients receiving the different TMD diagnoses, in order to gather as many data as possible on TMD epidemiology. To pursue the goal of an objective and standardized assessment of TMD patients, the Research Diagnostic Criteria for Temporomandibular Disorders (RDC/TMD) were proposed as guidelines for cross-center comparison of findings (Dworkin and Leresche 1992). Such a classification system is bi-axial, with an axis I evaluating the physical diagnoses and an axis II assessing the psychosocial issues, both providing specific and detailed diagnostic criteria. Despite their wide diffusion with multi-language translation and ongoing validation of revised diagnostic algorithms (Schifmann et al. 2010), a recent meta-analysis of the literature pointed out that only a few research groups actually described findings in their clinics' TMD patients populations by relying on the RDC/TMD (Manfredini et al. 2011c). From those studies, it emerged that myofascial pain was the most common diagnosis that combined muscle and joint disorders affect about half of the patients, and that different age peaks characterize subjects with disc displacement disorders with respect to those with inflammatory degenerative disorders (List et al. 1996; Winocur et al. 2009; Manfredini et al. 2010). Also, it emerged that the majority of TMD patients has psychosocial symptoms (i.e., psychological/psychiatric disorders related with a certain level of social impairment) belonging to the psychosocial sphere, as identified by the RDC/TMD axis II evaluating depression, somatization, and chronic pain-related impairment (Manfredini et al. 2011a).

Based on those premises, it seems to emerge that gathering more data on TMD patients populations is a compelling need to get deeper into the knowledge of disease epidemiology and to increase the external validity of the findings described so far, especially in the light of recent observations that a very low number of papers reported on both axis I and axis II findings (Palla 2011).

In consideration of the above need, the following strategy is provided as an example to describe the frequency of physical and psychosocial diagnoses in a sample of patients attending a TMD clinic (Manfredini et al. 2012a). The following sections on the description of the study design and report of main findings are thus based on an edited, arranged, and commented version of the manuscript "Manfredini et al. (2012a)".

2.2.2 Description of Study Sample and Design

When reporting epidemiological data, and more in general in all investigations involving populations of human subjects, it is always fundamental to present as much information as possible on the study population, in order to allow readers appraising the repeatability of the investigation and having a first glance at the representativeness of the study population. For instance, a sentence such as "Data were collected from 520 consecutive patients seeking treatment for TMD at the TMD Clinic, School of Dental Medicine, University of Pavia, during the period from January 1st 2006 to June 31st 2010." may be sufficiently exhaustive to introduce the study sample.

Then, details on the study design must be provided, with focus on the assessment procedures and the criteria for including/excluding subjects within the study population. Appropriate references must be provided for all procedures adopted in the investigation. In the case of an RDC/TMD-based epidemiological study, it should be specified that history taking and clinical examination were performed according to the RDC/TMD guidelines, and that, for instance, the standard, internationally accepted Italian version of the RDC/TMD instrument available since 2002 on the RDC/TMD consortium website was used by the authors to ease patients' comprehension. Criteria for exclusion are usually based on an age under 18 (due to the characteristics of the RDC/TMD, the reliability of which has been tested on adult populations), a concurrent diagnosis of other orofacial pain disorders, and presence of polyarthritis and/or other rheumatic disease. The focus on any specific diagnostic axis, viz., RDC/TMD axis I and/or II, should be mentioned. An important aspect of this kind of study design is that an epidemiological investigation should be based on widely adopted classification systems, thus avoiding any possible arbitrary authors' evaluation, which could reduce the internal and external validity of findings.

Once this premise was added to the study design, it often needs to provide some further details on the instruments adopted, since editors of peer-reviewed journals often ask for some additional specifications that allow readers to catch the main features of the diagnostic classification without referring to the original manuscript. So, it is important to give some information on the internal validity of the investigation, for instance by stating that all patients were simultaneously assessed by the same two examiners, who collected all RDC/TMD data and assigned axis I diagnoses by consensus. In the case of RDC/TMD, patients were given one or more of the following axis I group diagnoses: muscle disorders (group I), disc displacement (group II), and arthralgia, osteoarthritis, and osteoarthrosis (group III). As for axis II assessment, levels of depression and somatization were evaluated by the use of dedicated Symptoms Checklist-90 (SCL-90) items, while the Graded Chronic Pain Scale (GCPS) was used to rate pain-related impairment. Details on the diagnostic and scoring criteria were described in the original 1992 RDC/TMD publication (Dworkin and Leresche 1992).

A brief paragraph should then be dedicated to the ethical committee's approval and patients' consensus to take part to the study. Journals editors are facing an increasing demand for legal issues to be careful of, and sentences like "The investigation was based on routine clinical assessments and diagnostic activities of the TMD Clinic, with waiver from the local ethic committee. All patients gave their written informed consent to the clinical diagnostic procedures undertaken during the investigation and to the use of the so-gathered data for statistical purposes." are to be included in the materials and methods.

The final part of the study design section should present a description of the statistical/analytical approaches to data assessment and description. It is important that the statistical analyses are presented in details as for their need to answer any specific research questions. The order in which the statistical analyses are performed should be then followed exactly also in the results section of a manuscript, when the main findings of the investigation should be discussed on the basis of the same logical sequence. Of course, this general rule is much simpler in epidemiological studies than in other study designs. Indeed, for example, in the case of RDC/TMD findings in a population of TMD patients, most parts of the analyses are descriptive, and should be based on the report of the prevalence of the different RDC/TMD axis I diagnoses as well as the axis II psychosocial scores. Recent papers provided examples of how to stratify findings per age, to compare the age distribution of axis I and II diagnoses (Manfredini et al. 2012a). Then, ANOVA could be performed to test for the existence of differences in the mean age of diagnostic groups, with significance level set at $p < 0.05$. Importantly, if possible, the software with which all the statistical procedure were calculated should be indicated.

2.2.3   Description of Main Findings

In an epidemiological investigation on TMD patients, the main findings are basically represented by all kinds of possible information on the different diagnostic patterns and age distribution of the study subjects. The core results should be preceded by a specification of the number of patients who were excluded even if being potentially eligible for the study and the reasons for their exclusion. In the example of the above investigation (Manfredini et al. 2012a), all patients who were part of that consecutive sample but not satisfy the inclusion criteria should be listed in sentences as much detailed as possible, such as "$N=x$ patients were excluded from data analysis because of the following reasons: $N=x$ subjects received diagnoses of other orofacial pain disorders (i.e., atypical odontalgia), $N=x$ subjects had a concurrent diagnosis of fibromyalgia or other rheumatic disorders, and $N=x$ were aged under 18".

Then, the study findings should be reported in details, according to a structured sequence that may help readers following the strategy of reasoning adopted by the authors and catching the main messages (Table 2.1):

1. Number of patients satisfying inclusion criteria, for whom data are presented, with information on the sex distribution and mean age.
2. Frequency of each RDC/TMD axis I diagnostic subgroup, viz., group I disorders (muscle disorders), group II disorders (disc displacements), and group III disorders (arthralgia, osteoarthritis, and osteoarthrosis) in the study population. Of course, a table showing the distribution of specific RDC/TMD diagnoses should be fundamental to present the results in an intuitive way, especially to grasp data on the monolateral or bilateral disorders, which are seldom discussed in the TMD literature even if being fundamental issues in the clinical setting.
3. Frequency of axis I group diagnoses, alone or combined: muscle disorders alone, disc displacement disorders alone, arthralgia/arthrosis/arthritis, different combinations of group diagnoses.

Table 2.1 Example of a table showing the frequency of the different RDC/TMD axis I diagnoses in a sample of TMD patient population attending the University of Pavia ($N=462$ patients) Based on an edited version of the manuscript "Manfredini et al. (2012a)"

RDC/TMD axis I group diagnoses		Patients (N)	% frequency
I a—myofascial pain		169	36.5
I b—myofascial pain with limited opening		92	19.9
II a—disc displacement with reduction	R or L	102	22.0
	R and L	39	8.4
II b—disc displacement without reduction with limited opening	R or L	31	6.7
	R and L	7	1.5
II c—disc displacement without reduction without limited opening	R or L	9	1.9
	R and L	7	1.5
III a—arthralgia	R or L	123	26.6
	R and L	40	8.6
III b or III c—osteoarthritis/arthrosis	R or L	72	15.6
	R and L	31	6.7

R right joint, *L* left joint

4. Mean age of the patients receiving the different combinations of single and combined TMD diagnoses, with the aim to detect peculiar age patterns in diagnosis distribution (e.g., degenerative joint disorders are supposed to be more frequent in the older age groups). Also, for instance, some additional strategies to ascertain the age-related pattern of axis I diagnoses distribution could be performed, such as dividing the sample in various groups on the basis of percentile-derived intervals within the variable "age" and assessing the prevalence of different diagnoses in each age group.
5. Frequency and age distribution of the different axis II psychosocial disorders, viz., moderate or severe depression levels, moderate or severe somatization, different levels of pain-related impairment based on the Graded Chronic Pain Scale.

2.3 How to Test an Association Between Two Variables

2.3.1 Statement of the Problem

One of the main objectives of epidemiology is to define the etiological and risk factors for disease. In the field of TMD and orofacial pain, most studies on the etiology focused on the role of dental occlusion and bruxism. In particular, bruxism is commonly considered a major risk factor for TMD, but there are still many unsolved issues concerning the diagnosis of both disorders and their relationship (Svensson et al. 2008; Manfredini & Lobbezoo, 2010a). When introducing the issue of bruxism and TMD it should be pointed out since the early statements that the design of scientifically sound studies is complicated by difficulties in diagnosing clinical bruxism, as well as by the unclear relationship between instrumentally detected bruxism on the one hand and clinically diagnosed or self-perceived bruxism on the other hand. These difficulties also affect investigations on bruxism etiology and treatment, and a recent systematic review of the literature pointed out that inconsistent findings on the bruxism–TMD relationship may depend upon the adoption of non-homogeneous diagnostic techniques among studies (Manfredini and Lobbezoo 2010b). Works on self-reported or clinical bruxism diagnosis commonly showed a positive association with TMD pain, while, on the contrary, such positive association was not always confirmed with studies using instrumental bruxism detection, viz., by means of polysomnography (PSG) and/or electromyography (EMG). Also, the studies on the bruxism–TMD relationship rarely relied on standardized TMD diagnoses.

Based on those controversies, a possible strategy to ease the comparison of findings is to adopt standardized and reproducible diagnostic procedures for both TMD and bruxism. Thus, as in the case of epidemiological investigations, such purpose could be achieved with the diffusion of information gained over the years with the RDC/TMD, which, as stated above, provides diagnostic guidelines for TMDs as well as an anamnestic investigation of awake and sleep bruxism (Dworkin and Leresche 1992). Until recent years, no studies addressed the issues of the prevalence of TMD and bruxism by relying on the RDC/TMD for diagnosing both disorders, and a multicenter study was thus performed at two highly specialized centers for the treatment of bruxism, TMD, and orofacial pain (Manfredini et al. 2012c), with the aims: (1) to report the frequency of TMD diagnoses and prevalence of self-reported awake and sleep bruxism in patient populations recruited at two highly specialized clinics; and (2) to describe the possible differences between findings of the two centers as a basis to suggest recommendations for future improvements in diagnostic homogeneity and accuracy. The following sections on the description of the study design and report of main findings in the case of an investigation assessing the association between two variables are thus based on an edited, arranged, and commented version of the manuscript "Manfredini et al. (2012c)".

2.3.2   Description of Study Sample and Design

As in the case of epidemiological studies and also in all example investigations described throughout the book, as much information as possible on the study design should be provided. For instance, it is important to describe if the study is prospective/longitudinal or retrospective. The latter design allows drawing no conclusions on the cause–effect relationship between the variables under investigation, but is the most diffuse strategy to gather data on large samples for obvious reasons of study feasibility. In the case of a multicenter study, all details of the clinical records of the samples of patients and their recruitment modalities should be reported. The importance of reporting data in accordance to the RDC/TMD guidelines and the version(s) used has been discussed in details in the above example of epidemiological study.

Importantly, in the case of bruxism–TMD investigations, the RDC/TMD's standardized history taking should be used to record data on self-reported awake and sleep bruxism, on the basis of the patients' answers to questions 15c ("Do you clench or grind your teeth during sleep?") and 15d ("Do you clench or grind your teeth while awake?"). For a detailed description of the diagnostic criteria, it is always important to refer to the original RDC/TMD publication (Dworkin and Leresche 1992) and to the successive studies (Truelove et al. 2010), some of which have raised concerns that have been taken into consideration when revising the current RDC/TMD guidelines (Steenks and de Wijer 2009; Anderson et al. 2010; Lobbezoo et al. 2010).

In the case of retrospective studies, the strategies for gathering patients' databases must be reported also in terms of the time span during which the patient populations were recruited. This issue assumes importance and must be discussed in detail in some particular conditions when the time spans for collecting data on the various populations are different across the centers involved in the multicenter investigation. In the example paper reporting a multicenter study on the bruxism–TMD relationship (Manfredini et al. 2012c), patients attending the TMD Clinic of the University of Padova, Italy, were recruited during the period from January 1, 2009 to June 31, 2009, while those attending the Orofacial Pain Clinic of the University of Tel Aviv, Israel, were recruited more than 5 years before, during the period from January 1, 2001 to December 31, 2004. Despite both centers being served as reference clinics for patients' referral from vast areas around their location, and investigators responsible for the RDC/TMD assessments have been involved in previous publications on RDC/TMD-related epidemiological and diagnostic issues (Manfredini and Guarda-Nardini 2008; Winocur et al. 2009), the risk for non-homogeneity of data between the two centers should be taken into proper account and discussed thoroughly. In both clinics, several examiners were involved in the diagnostic process, data gathering, and treatment planning, but the final supervision for each single patient's RDC/TMD diagnosis belonged to the clinicians who were responsible for the projects, as to increase the internal validity of findings. In any case, it is fundamental that findings of the various centers are also presented separately.

From a statistical viewpoint, such kind of investigation is constituted by two strategies:

1. Descriptive reports of the prevalence of each of the single and multiple RDC/TMD axis I diagnoses for TMDs as well as the frequency of positive answers to the questions on self-reported bruxism.
2. Comparison between the two centers of the frequency of the different combinations of clinical TMD diagnoses (no diagnoses; myofascial pain; disc displacement; inflammatory–degenerative joint disorders; myofascial pain and disc displacement; myofascial pain and inflammatory–degenerative joint disorders; disc displacement and inflammatory–degenerative joint disorders; myofascial pain, disc displacement, and inflammatory–degenerative joint disorders) and anamnestical bruxism reports (no reported bruxism; reported awake clenching/grinding; reported sleep clenching/grinding; reported awake and sleep clenching/grinding).

Table 2.2 Example of a cross-tabulation of RDC/TMD diagnosis and self-reported bruxism diagnosis in a sample of TMD patients recruited at the University of Padova, Italy ($N=219$). Values are expressed in percentage and refer to the total of the patients receiving each specific diagnosis. Based on an edited version of the manuscript "Manfredini et al. (2012c)"

	No SR bruxism	Awake	Asleep	Awake and asleep
No TMD	80	0	0	20
Myofascial pain alone	38.1	23.8	9.5	28.5
Disc displacement alone	60	20	0	20
Inflammatory–degenerative disorders alone	62.5	9.5	12.3	15.7
Myofascial pain + disc displacement	33.3	0	33.3	33.3
Myofascial pain + inflammatory– degenerative disorders	48.3	13.5	16.7	21.5
Disc displacement + inflammatory– degenerative disorders	66.6	2.7	13.8	21.9
Myofascial pain + disc displacement + inflammatory–degenerative disorders	52.1	13	13	21.9

MP myofascial pain, *DD* disc displacement, *IDD* inflammatory–degenerative disorders, *SR* self-report

2.3.3 Description of Main Findings

Since the strategies for reporting epidemiological findings have been already discussed, focus in the below lines will be on the cross-centers comparison and the bruxism–TMD association. The above multicenter investigation showed significant differences, which were shown between the two clinic samples as for the frequency of TMD diagnoses, with myofascial pain alone being the most prevalent diagnosis in the Tel Aviv sample and myofascial pain combined with inflammatory–degenerative disorders in Padova. A chi-square test showed that the distribution of the different RDC/TMD diagnoses was significantly different between the two centers, and the authors are always recommended to present the level of significance (e.g., chi-square, $p<0.001$) in the text and tables. If possible, gender-related diagnoses' distribution should also be presented.

The same information must be provided on bruxism items, with the percentage of positive endorsement to the RDC/TMD questions 15c ("sleep clenching/grinding") and/or 15d ("awake clenching/grinding"). Again, the frequency of answers should be recorded separately between the two centers (e.g., percentage of subjects answering "yes" to at least one of the two bruxism items in the Tel Aviv and in the Padova sample), with an appropriate statistical comparison (e.g., chi-square test is enough for such comparison in the majority of situations).

Importantly, the prevalence of self-reported bruxism in the different TMD diagnostic groups, which represents the main target of the study, should be reported for all the patient populations. In the example multicenter investigation, in the Tel Aviv population patients with myofascial pain alone tended to report bruxism more frequently than patients receiving other diagnoses, while in the Padova sample the prevalence of self-reported bruxism was similar among the different TMD diagnostic groups (Table 2.2).

2.4   How to Assess the Amount of Variance for Disease Explained by an Etiological Model

The above bruxism–TMD investigation provided an example of a single variable association/correlation analysis (i.e., the presence of a variable (bruxism) is used to predict the presence of the other variable (TMD)), which is a statistical approach that is not suitable to depict the multifactorial biological models at best. More complex examples of studies investigating the role of etiological/risk factors for disease are based on analyses in which more than one variable are used as predictors of the outcome variable, viz., the presence of disease. Such an approach provided that the role of each single predictor is influenced by the concurrent presence/absence of the other predictors, and it is called multiple variable analysis. Historically, the most interesting multiple variable studies in the field of TMD and orofacial pain came from investigations assessing the role of dental occlusion features as risk factors for bruxism and TMD.

To introduce the issue, it must be recognized that the etiology of bruxism, as it happens with TMD, is one of the most debated issues in dentistry. Past theories on the purported role of dental occlusion abnormalities in the etiology of bruxism have never been proven, and they have progressively lost importance in favor of theories supporting the role of other factors of central origin (e.g., psychosocial, neurobiological, and genetic factors) (Lavigne et al. 2008). In general, the recent literature suggests a shift from occlusal to psychological-based hypotheses and from peripheral to central regulation hypotheses (Lobbezoo and Naeije 2001; Lobbezoo et al. 2012). Notwithstanding that, the hypothesis that certain occlusal features may be related with bruxism onset has not been completely abandoned and is occasionally revisited (Sugimoto et al. 2011).

Actually, for a causal relationship between occlusion and bruxism being present, a compelling prerequisite is that the two variables are associated, viz., the prevalence of the disorder should be significantly higher in subjects presenting a certain risk factor (Hill 1965; Manfredini and Lobbezoo 2010a). Only then, hypothesis-driven studies to test the existence of a causal link may be performed on a rational basis. Past works on the issue showed that an association between bruxism and occlusal features of the natural dentition could be ruled out (Lobbezoo et al. 2001; Manfredini et al. 2004) and, in general, comprehensive reviews on the argument suggested that bruxism and the bite are likely unrelated (Lobbezoo et al. 2012). Nonetheless, the quality of the available literature on the argument is not optimal, and it might be interesting to get deeper into the issue by the adoption of the above-introduced multiple variable analyses of the various occlusal risk factors, which is more apt to depict biological models.

Within these premises, some characteristics of a recent investigation aiming to estimate the contribution of various occlusal features of the natural dentition to identify self-reported bruxers with respect to non-bruxers can be used as example to guide readers through the multiple variable assessment of risk for disease (Manfredini et al. 2012b). The following sections on the description of the study design and report of main findings in the case of an investigation assessing the association between two variables in a multifactorial model are thus based on an edited, arranged, and commented version of the manuscript "Manfredini et al. (2012b)."

2.4.1   Description of Study Sample and Design

As usual, details on the study subjects must be provided, and it is interesting to point out that in this particular case patients with orofacial pain were excluded from the study sample due to the possible influence of the presence of pain on the relation between the predictor variables, viz., dental occlusion features, and the variable to be predicted, viz., bruxism. This choice was particularly smart by the authors, and such an approach should be recommended in all cases that "pure" samples are needed to assess the relationship between the factors under investigation.

This kind of study should be usually performed according to a case-control design, with age- and sex-matched groups of cases (e.g., self-reported bruxers) and controls (e.g., self-reported non-bruxers). If possible, it is important that both samples were recruited among the same population (e.g., patients attending a dental school for conservative care). As usual, details should be provided on the diagnostic strategies. For instance, the presence of bruxism is usually anamnestically investigated based on self-reported clenching and/or grinding of the teeth during the day and/or the night. In the field of dentistry, much focus is always put also on the definition of the occlusal features that should be recorded for each patient, since their definition is not always the same for the different dental specialties (e.g., orthodontics, prosthetic dentistry, conservative dentistry). For an orofacial pain practitioner, suffice is to state that, for example, retruded contact position (RCP) to intercuspal contact position (ICP) slide length (<2 mm was considered normal), vertical overlap (<0 mm was considered an anterior open bite; >4 mm, a deep bite), horizontal overlap (>4 mm was considered a large horizontal overlap), incisor dental midline discrepancy (<2 mm was considered normal), the presence of a unilateral posterior cross-bite, mediotrusive interferences, and laterotrusive interferences, were recorded through a clinical examination that was made by the same trained operator.

As for the statistical design, an interesting strategy is to perform first a single variable analysis to identify the potentially significant associations between the occlusal predictors and bruxism. Then, those variables that at single variable analysis reached a significance level under an arbitrary cutoff value (e.g., $p < 0.10$) could be included in a multiple variable regression model in which one predictor controls for the others. An alternative approach should be to include all variables in the regression model, but the former approach should be preferred to avoid a sort of "fishing expedition" without any logical premises. Based on the above, a suitable design for the occlusion–bruxism assessment should be to compare the prevalence of the assessed occlusal features in self-reported bruxers and in non-bruxers by means of single regression analysis. Values of sensitivity, specificity, positive predictive values (PPV) and negative predictive values (NPV), and accuracy to detect self-reported bruxism were assessed on the basis of 2×2 contingency tables (rows: occlusal features; columns: bruxism). PPV and NPV were calculated on the basis of the bruxism prevalence in this study's group, while accuracy was defined as the percentage of subjects which were correctly classified by the presence of each single occlusal feature. Subsequently, a multiple logistic regression model was used to identify the significant associations between the assessed occlusal features (independent variables) and self-reported bruxism (dependent variable). Only those factors that were significant at $p < 0.10$ in the single regression analysis were included in the initial multiple regression model. Then, the variable with the weakest association with "recovery" was removed from the multiple regression model. This was repeated in a backward stepwise manner until all variables that were retained in the model showed a $p \leq 0.05$. The odds ratios (OR) for bruxism were assessed for each occlusal variable, while simultaneously controlling for the other variables in the model. OR values higher than 2 are commonly considered significant from a clinical viewpoint. Nagelkerke's R-square (R^2) was obtained as an estimation of the total variance explained by the occlusal factors included in the model. If R^2 is > 0.75, the regression model is considered capable to predict the presence of disease at a very good level. The model's ability to predict disease is considered good if R^2 is comprised between 0.50 and 0.75, fair if R^2 is comprised between 0.25 and 0.50, and poor for a R^2 of 0.25 or less (Cox and Snell 1989). The accuracy of the final logistic regression model to predict bruxer (sensitivity) or non-bruxer (specificity) status as well as PPV and NPV were determined from a 2×2 classification table.

2.4.2   Description of Main Findings

Based on the above strategy, findings should be reported according to the same sequence of analyses:

1. A comparison of the prevalence of the assessed occlusal features in self-reported bruxers and non-bruxers was performed by means of single regression analysis to build a multiple regression, with detailed description of the level of each specific association that was retrieved. Also, accuracy values to predict self-reported bruxism by means of single predictors should be reported (Table 2.3).
2. In the case of the example study design, the three variables showing a $p < 0.10$ (slide ≥ 2 mm; mediotrusive interferences; laterotrusive interferences) were entered in the multiple regression model, and the variable remaining in the final model was laterotrusive interferences. This means that the data on the mediotrusive interferences and slide did not add any information to the regression model including laterotrusive interferences ($p = 0.030$). Laterotrusive interferences showed an OR for self-reported bruxism of about 2.6. The percentage of explained variance for bruxism by the final multiple regression model was 4.6 % (Nagelkerke's $R^2 = 0.046$). This model including only one occlusal factor showed unacceptable PPV (58.1 %) and NPV (59.7 %), thus showing a poor accuracy to predict the presence of self-reported bruxism (59.2 %).

In conclusion, the above study design allowed showing that the amount of variance for bruxism that was explained by the various occlusal features was low. In other words, the role of dental occlusion as a risk factor for bruxism was minimal and not relevant in the clinical setting.

Table 2.3 Comparison of the prevalence of the occlusal features in self-reported bruxers and controls, and significance in the single regression analysis. Accuracy, specificity, sensitivity, PPV, and NPV of single occlusal features to predict self-reported bruxism are also reported. Data based on findings from a recent study, edited version of the manuscript "Manfredini et al. (2012b)"

Variables	Bruxers	Controls	Sig.	Odds ratio (95 % C.I.)	Accuracy (%)	Specificity (%)	Sensitivity (%)	PPV (%)	NPV (%)
Laterotrusive interferences	19/67	10/75	0.030	2.57 (1.09–6.03)	59.1	89.3	28.3	65.5	57.5
Mediotrusive interferences	31/67	22/75	0.037	2.07 (1.03–4.14)	59.1	70.6	46.2	58.4	59.5
Anterior open-bite	1/4	3/75	0.367	0.36 (0.03–3.58)	51.4	96	1.5	25	52.1
Unilateral cross-bite	18/67	17/75	0.562	0.79 (0.37–1.71)	53.5	77.3	26.8	51.4	54.2
Large horizontal overlap	4/67	9/75	0.214	0.46 (0.13–1.58)	49.2	88	5.9	30.7	51.1
Dental midline discrepancy	26/67	33/75	0.531	1.23 (0.63–2.42)	47.8	56	38.8	44.1	50.6
Deep-bite	20/67	17/75	0.330	1.45 (0.68–3.08)	54.9	77.3	29.8	54	55.2
Slide RCP–ICP>2 mm	23/67	16/75	0.083	0.51 (0.24–1.09)	57.7	78.6	34.3	58.9	56.7

2.5   How to Assess the Correlation between Continuous Variables

In the clinical and research settings, the search for valid diagnostic approaches to bruxism has been always an argument for debate, and it was suggested that consistency of findings from the bruxism literature can be increased with the adoption of standardized techniques to record masticatory muscle activity (MMA). Indeed, bruxism is not a disorder per se, and may be viewed as a physiopathological continuum, since about 60 % of asymptomatic subjects reportedly shows signs of rhythmic MMA during sleep (Lavigne et al. 2008). Moreover, due to the difficulties to find adequately equipped sleep laboratories and to the potential bias related with a laboratory-based diagnostic approach, it seems plausible to hypothesize that the use of portable EMG home-recording devices may be a promising strategy to increase knowledge on the issue. Of course, when linear measures such as the amplitude of EMG signals are assessed, all attempts to define cutoffs for dichotomize outcome variable into a categorical one are arbitrary, and statistical approaches that are suitable for depicting the relationship between continuous variables are needed.

Within these premises, the number of studies adopting measurements approaches to bruxism diagnosis is increasing both in the field of etiological and treatment studies. To get deeper into the issue of the study designs, an example study may be a recent investigation attempting to describe the correlation between sleep-time MMA and psychological symptoms by the use of an EMG home-recording device in a group of healthy volunteers completing a battery of psychometric questionnaires (Manfredini et al. 2011b). The following sections on the description of the study design and report of main findings in the case of an investigation assessing the correlation between two continuous variables are thus based on an edited, arranged, and commented version of the manuscript Manfredini et al. (2011b).

2.5.1   Description of Study Sample and Design

From a methodological viewpoint, it must be pointed out that this kind of investigation should be ideally performed in asymptomatic volunteers to avoid the potential influence of confounding factors (e.g., pain) on the relationship between the two variables for which the level of association is under testing, viz., bruxism and psychosocial factors. Based on this need, a standardized psychiatric instrument should be used for the exclusion of clinically evident mental diseases. It should be also remarked that experimental protocols of bruxism measurements are at risk of subjects' dropout from the protocol; thus, details on the number of subjects dropping out from the study and the reasons for their withdrawal have to be carefully listed to take into proper account for the percentage of failed recording nights.

Details of the study design should be carefully described. In the example investigation on bruxism and psychosocial factors, each subject underwent one night of electromyographic recording, with the concurrent evaluation of four different muscles (bilateral masseter and anterior temporalis muscles). The sleep-related

EMG recording was preceded by the completion of a battery of validated psycho-metric tests and by the recording of a brief EMG track to set the home-recording device for the detection of cutoff values. While the attempt to measure the activity of all four main masticatory muscles as well as the choice of the appropriate psychometric instruments were major strengths, the single-night recording was a study limitation because of the lack of information on the night-to-night variability of the EMG activity. In similar situations, the authors have the duty to recognize and discuss their study's limits, and the journal readers and/or reviewers must always appraise the "unbiased" way the authors present their data.

Experimental studies often featured ad hoc instruments that need to be described in detail. For instance, an innovative portable device to record masseter and temporalis muscles activity bilaterally was designed for use in the above investigation. Four out of the 16 channels supported by the EMG recorder were used (right and left masseter and temporalis muscles); signals were amplified and digitalized at a sampling frequency of 1,000 Hz (with a 16 bit A/D resolution). Technical characteristics were optimal as far as the hardware and software components were concerned, but the home recording of four muscles' activity was so complicated that such an investigation still remains unique in its kind.

One interesting feature of the study design was the authors' choice of the cutoff values (average muscle activity of the three attempts) for the non-functional muscle activities. At the beginning of each recording session, the subjects performed three swallowing movements to set such a cutoff, viz., the EMG activity recorded during swallowing was considered as the higher extreme of function and all EMG events above that activity were considered as markers of nonfunctional muscle activity. Such an interesting choice, again unique in its kind, was based on literature data showing that EMG activity of the masseter muscles during swallowing might be discriminated from those recorded during other activities in 90 % of cases (Gallo et al. 1998), thus providing a theoretical and practical support to the use of such parameter to create a threshold for the detection of the nonfunctional EMG events.

The software was set to automatically detect any EMG event with a higher amplitude with respect to the root-mean-squared (RMS) amplitude recorded with swallowing movements. Because sleep variables were not scored and other higher-than-swallow amplitude confounding orofacial activities like apnea/hypopnea and sleep talking cannot be identified on the basis of EMG alone, the data could not be interpreted strictly in terms of sleep bruxism behavior. Therefore, in line with previous studies adopting EMG alone (Van Selms et al. 2008) and using unspecific terms, in that investigation the generic term sleep-time MMA was used (Manfredini et al. 2011b). For each muscle, the total MMA duration (in seconds) during the 5-hour span and per each 1-hour increment was assessed. The integrated EMG signal was adopted to quantify the work produced by each muscle ($\mu V \times sec$) during the 5-hour span and per each 1-hour increment.

In brief, all theoretical and technical issues concerning the study design as well as its limitations were carefully described by the authors, which were smartly guided and advised by the editor and reviewers through the publication process, thus providing a good framework to appraise the validity of the investigation and improve its readability.

As for the statistical approach, descriptive data were calculated for each of the main study variables, viz., psychometric scores and parameters related to muscle activity. A t test was run to compare means between each pair of symmetric muscles, and right and left data were pooled together for statistical analysis. Correlations between the MMA duration (total and per each 1-hour increment) for masseter and temporalis muscles and scores endorsed in the psychometric instruments were tested with Pearson's test. Linear backward regression models were created to identify predictors of muscle work for masseter and temporalis muscles, by the adoption of parameters related to EMG data (muscle work ($\mu V \times sec$) during the 5-hour span and during each 1-hour increment) as dependent variables, while total scores obtained in the psychometric tests (STAI-X, STAXI, BDI-II) were considered independent variables. As usual, statistical significance was set at $p < 0.05$.

2.5.2   Description of Main Findings

Such an investigation, and in general all experimental/laboratory studies, provided an huge amount of data for discussion, and the authors should be able to present them in a logical order, starting with some general considerations on the scores in the various psychometric measures and going deeper with the analysis of MMA data and their relationship with an individual's psychometric scores.

The average total number of MMA events as well as their duration during the 5-hour recording period were presented for each muscle. Importantly, the differences between each pair of right and left muscles were not statistically significant. The absence of difference in the pair of muscles allowed the authors to pool together EMG data for paired muscles to assess the resulting muscle work ($\mu V \times sec$), which was mainly related to the temporalis muscles in every 1-hour increment. The amount of muscle work produced by the right and left temporalis muscles was variable within the 5-hour span and ranged between 1.58 and 2.25 $\mu V \times s$, while the work produced by the masseter muscles was lower, within the 0.75–1.03 $\mu V \times s$ range. The total amount of muscle work of the four muscles during the whole recording period was in average 13.5 $\mu V \times s$. Correlation analysis for continuous variables showed that trait anxiety scores were significantly correlated to the total amount of MMA duration (in seconds) of the temporalis muscles ($r = 0.558$; $p = 0.031$). The authors then went into more details, reporting that the duration of MMA events during the first hour of recording was related to trait anxiety scores for both temporalis ($r = 0.584$; $p = 0.022$) and masseter muscles ($r = 0.660$; $p = 0.007$). The most important finding that was detected by means of the analysis was that, while the significant correlation between MMA duration in temporalis muscles and trait anxiety was detected also in the second hour increment ($r = 0.676$; $p = 0.006$), the correlation between trait anxiety and muscles' activity got progressively lost in the following hours. No significant correlations emerged between the duration of MMA and scores endorsed in the other psychometric instruments. Subjects with high trait anxiety scores, viz., higher than the median value, had a significantly higher temporalis muscles MMA duration in the first 3 hour increments and masseter muscles MMA duration in the first recording hour with respect to low-anxiety traits subjects.

Regression analysis showed that the total amount of work produced by the four muscles during the 5-hour span was unrelated to any of the psychometric scores. Significant relationship did emerge between STAI-T ($p=0.038$) scores and work produced during the first recording hour ($R^2=0.408$). STAI-T scores ($p=0.013$), along with BDI scores ($p=0.014$), were also related to the second-hour work ($R^2=0.471$). No other significant psychometric predictors were identified for any of the other 1-hour increments.

In summary, such a detailed study design allowed showing for the first time in the orofacial pain literature that the duration of sleep-time MMA, especially during the early phases of a night's sleep, may be related to anxiety trait, and not to anxiety state, depression, or anger. These findings may support the view that features related with the individual management of anxiety, viz., trait, are likely to be more important than acute episodes of anxiety, viz., state, in the etiology of sleep-time MMA. The role of other psychological symptoms is likely to be less important.

References

Anderson GC, Gonzalez YM, Ohrbach R, Truelove EL, Sommers E, Look JO, Schiffman EL. The research diagnostic criteria for temporomandibular disorders. VI. Future directions. J Orofac Pain. 2010; 24:79–88.

Cox DR, Snell EJ. Analysis of binary data. 2nd ed. London: Chapman and Hall; 1989. p. 209.

Dworkin S, LeResche L. Research diagnostic criteria for temporomandibular disorders: review, criteria examinations and specifications, critique. J Craniomandib Disord Fac Oral Pain. 1992; 6:301–55.

Gallo LM, Guerra PO, Palla S. Automatic on-line one-channel recognition of masseter activity. J Dent Res. 1998; 77:1539–46.

Hill BA. The environment and disease: association or causation? Proc Royal Soc Med. 1965; 58:295–300.

Lavigne GJ, Khoury S, Abe S, Yamaguchi T, Raphael K. Bruxism physiology and pathology: an overview for clinicians. J Oral Rehabil. 2008; 35:476–94.

List T, Dworkin SF. Comparing TMD diagnoses and clinical findings at Swedish and US TMD centers using research diagnostic criteria for temporomandibular disorders. J Orofac Pain. 1996;10:240–53.

Lobbezoo F, Naeije M. Bruxism is mainly regulated centrally, not peripherally. J Oral Rehabil. 2001; 28:1085–91.

Lobbezoo F, Visscher CM, Naeije M. Some remarks on the RDC/TMD validation project: report of an IADR/Toronto-2008 workshop discussion. J Oral Rehabil. 2010; 37:779–83.

Lobbezoo F, Rompré PH, Soucy JP, Iafrancesco C, Turkewicz J, Montplaisir JY, Lavigne GJ. Lack of associations between occlusal and cephalometric measures, side imbalance in striatal D2 receptor binding, and sleep-related oromotor activities. J Orofac Pain. 2001; 15:64–73.

Lobbezoo F, Ahlberg J, Manfredini D, Winocur E. Are bruxism and the bite causally related? J Oral Rehabil. 2012; 39:489–501.

Manfredini D, Guarda-Nardini L. Agreement between research diagnostic criteria for temporomandibular disorders and magnetic resonance diagnoses of temporomandibular disc displacement in a patients population. Int J Oral Maxillofac Surg. 2008; 37:612–6.

Manfredini D, Lobbezoo F. Bruxism and temporomandibular disorders. In: Manfredini D, Editor. Current concepts on temporomandibular disorders. Berlin: Quintessence Publishing; 2010a. p. 135–52.

Manfredini D, Lobbezoo F. Relationship between bruxism and temporomandibular disorders: a systematic review of literature from 1998 to 2008. Oral Surg Oral Med Oral Pathol Oral Radiol Endod. 2010b; 109:e26–e50.

Manfredini D, Landi N, Tognini F, Montagnani G, Bosco M. Occlusal features are not a reliable predictor of bruxism. Minerva Stomatol 2004;53:231–9.

Manfredini D, Piccotti F, Ferronato G, Guarda-Nardini L. Age peaks of different RDC/TMD diagnoses in a patient population. J Dent. 2010; 38:392–9.

Manfredini D, Ahlberg J, Winocur E, Guarda-Nardini L, Lobbezoo F. Correlation of RDC/TMD axis I diagnoses and axis II pain-related disability. A multicenter study. Clin Oral Investig. 2011a; 15:749–56.

Manfredini D, Fabbri A, Peretta R, Guarda-Nardini L, Lobbezoo F. Influence of psychological symptoms on home-recorded sleep-time masticatory muscle activity in healthy subjects. J Oral Rehabil. 2011b; 38:902–11.

Manfredini D, Guarda-Nardini L, Winocur E, Piccotti F, Ahlberg J, Lobbezoo F. Research diagnostic criteria for temporomandibular disorders: a systematic review of axis I epidemiologic findings. Oral Surg Oral Med Oral Pathol Oral Radiol Endod. 2011c; 112:453–62.

Manfredini D, Arveda N, Guarda-Nardini L, Segù M, Collesano V. Distribution of diagnoses in a TMD patient population. Oral Surg Oral Med Oral Pathol Oral Radiol Endod. 2012a; 114:e35–e41.

Manfredini D, Visscher C, Guarda-Nardini L, Lobbezoo F. Occlusal factors are not related with self-reported bruxism. J Orofac Pain. 2012b; 26:163–7.

Manfredini D, Winocur E, Guarda-Nardini L, Lobbezoo F. Self-reported bruxism and temporomandibular disorders. Findings from two specialised centers. J Oral Rehabil. 2012c; 39:319–25.

Palla S. Biopsychosocial pain model crippled? J Orofac Pain. 2011; 25:289–90.

Rollmann GB, Gillespie JM. The role of psychosocial factors in temporomandibular disorders. Curr Rev Pain. 2000; 4:71–81.

Schiffman EL, Ohrbach R, Truelove EL, Tai F, Anderson GC, Pan W, et al. The research diagnostic criteria for temporomandibular disorders. V: methods used to establish and validate revised axis I diagnostic algorithms. J Orofac Pain. 2010; 24:63–78.

Steenks MH, de Wijer A. Validity of the research diagnostic criteria for temporomandibular disorders axis I in clinical and research settings. J Orofac Pain. 2009; 23:9–16.

Sugimoto K, Yoshimi H, Sasaguri K, Sato S. Occlusion factors influencing the magnitude of sleep bruxism activity. Cranio. 2011; 29:127–37.

Suvinen TI, Reade PC, Kemppainen P, Kononen M, Dworkin SF. Review of aetiological concepts of temporomandibular pain disorders: a biopsychosocial model for integration of physical disorder factors with psychological and psychosocial illness impact factors. Eur J Pain. 2005; 9:613–33.

Svensson P, Jadidi F, Arima T, Baad-Hansen L, Sessle BJ. Relationships between craniofacial pain and bruxism. J Oral Rehabil. 2008; 35:524–47.

Truelove E, Pan W, Look JO, Mancl LA, Ohrbach RK, Velly AM, Huggins KH, Lenton P, Schiffman EL. The research diagnostic criteria for temporomandibular disorders. III: validity of axis I diagnoses. J Orofac Pain. 2010; 24:35–47.

Van Selms MK, Lobbezoo F, Visscher CM, Naeije M. Myofascial temporomandibular disorder pain, parafunctions and psychological stress. J Oral Rehabil. 2008; 35:45–52.

Winocur E, Steinkeller-Dekel M, Reiter S, Eli I. A retrospective analysis of temporomandibular findings among Israeli-born patients based on the RDC/TMD. J Oral Rehabil. 2009; 36:11–7.

Chapter 3
Diagnosis and Treatment

Luca Guarda-Nardini, Rosa Arboretti and Daniele Manfredini

The present chapter covers a wide spectrum of topics related with the diagnosis and treatment of TMD. As in the case of the previous section on the epidemiology and etiology, some example investigations were chosen in the attempt to keep the readers updated with the current clinical, and not only statistical, concepts on TMD practice. In the field of diagnosis, interesting methodological strategies to discuss were found in the literature on TMJ imaging, which is suitable to provide examples on how to test diagnostic accuracy of less-frequently adopted imaging techniques such as ultrasonography (US), as well as in the studies on instrumental devices, which example the way some common beliefs did not pass the filter of evidence. In the field of treatment, some studies by the authors' research group were commented to illustrate some of the different kind of investigations that can be performed and the possible approaches that can be adopted to design a research protocol. In these specific cases, the authors' experience with TMJ arthrocentesis and injections protocols is used as a starting point to comment on the different study design and, despite not being fully representative of the full spectrum of treatment modalities in the field of TMD and orofacial pain, it provides an evidence-based framework for reading and designing investigations on TMD treatment.

L. Guarda-Nardini (✉) · R. Arboretti · D. Manfredini
University of Padova, Padova, Italy
e-mail: luca.guarda@unipd.it

R. Arboretti
e-mail: rosa.arboretti@unipd.it

D. Manfredini
e-mail: daniele.manfredini@tin.it

L. Salmaso et al., *Statistical Approaches to Orofacial Pain and Temporomandibular Disorders Research*, SpringerBriefs in Statistics, DOI 10.1007/978-1-4939-0876-9_3,
© The Author(s) 2014

Table 3.1 Characteristics of an ideal diagnostic instrument or approach. The higher the values in all the characteristics, the higher the chance that the diagnosis is correct

Characteristics of a diagnostic instrument/approach	
Reliability	The instrument gives the same result when the test is performed by different examiners (inter-examiner reliability) or by the same examiner at different times (intra-operator reliability)
Sensitivity	The instrument detects all the subjects with the disease
Specificity	The instrument detects all the healthy subjects
Predictive value	The results are indicative of the actual presence (positive predictive value, PPV) or absence (negative predictive value, NPV) of the disease
Accuracy	The instrument provides a measure which is correct in average
Validity	The results are clinically useful

3.1   The Need to Detect Diagnostic Accuracy and Define Treatment Effectiveness

Typically, the path to diagnose a disease provides that the clinician elaborates a working hypothesis to be tested against alternative hypotheses, viz., a process of differential diagnosis, by means of instruments providing the best available diagnostic accuracy, viz., confirmative test. Thus, the final diagnosis is usually the result of a hypotheti-codeductive process that, starting with the recording of the patient's anamnesis and chief complaints, leads to the construction of a diagnostic hypothesis that is based on the clinician's knowledge, experience, and expertise. Once the process of critical thinking that leads to the diagnostic hypothesis is performed, the diagnostic process follows a path, which is commonly described in specialist orofacial pain textbooks (Goulet and Palla 2008; Manfredini 2010).

Ideally, the diagnostic process is simplified in the case of diseases for which an accurate diagnosis is possible by means of instruments or assessment techniques that provide reliable and valid information, based on one instrument's capability to detect the main symptoms of a disease (Table 3.1).

In the case of TMD, and orofacial pain conditions in general, the possibility to build up this process is questionable due to the multifactorial etiology of the disease, and the possibility to define highly accurate diagnostic instruments is limited by the fact the main clinical marker for treatment need is the presence of pain. Thus, any diagnostic device or technique should stand comparison with a clinical assessment of the complex pain experience, which can be viewed as the target of reference for TMD diagnosis.

As for treatment, interesting data came from studies assessing the prevalence of treatment-demanding TMD. In particular, a recent meta-analysis of treatment need for TMD in adult non-patients showed that very few data exist on this issue and that only 17 papers in the history of the TMD literature have estimated the prevalence of treatment need (Al-Jundi et al. 2008). Those papers came from very few longitudinal researches conducted by few research groups, mostly located in Scandinavian universities, thus limiting generalizability of results. The estimated prevalence of treatment need for TMD in adults is about 16%.

The need for TMD treatment has to be based on precise indications related to the presence of pain, severe limitations in jaw function, and/or signs of degenerative diseases of the TMJ. Besides, there are some clinical signs or associated features that, in the absence of consistent positive or negative evidence of their relationship with the onset of treatment-demanding TMD symptoms, has to be addressed independently by the presence of TMD, such as tooth grinding and jaw clenching, or considered potential risk factors to be assessed at the individual level, such as disc displacement. Such signs and symptoms may be the clinical manifestations of different underlying diseases, the etiology and pathophysiology of which can be seldom identified, thus making causal therapy hard to achieve in the majority of cases. For these reasons, TMD treatment should be delivered mainly in the form of patients' management, viz., symptomatic treatment, with the obvious notable exceptions of some surgery-demanding conditions. The armamentarium of the TMD practitioner is made of many conservative and reversible therapeutic modalities, such as physiotherapy and physical treatments, drugs, cognitive–behavioral approaches, some types of oral appliances, TMJ arthrocentesis, and intra-articular injections of medications, which seem to be all supported by a valid rationale for use and good treatment effectiveness.

Based on these premises, and considering the difficulties to define diagnostic accuracy and treatment effectiveness in pain patients, examples of different study designs to get deeper into the diagnosis and treatment of TMD will be provided in the remaining section of this chapter.

3.2   How to Assess Diagnostic Accuracy with Dichotomic Variables: Agreement Between Two Techniques and Predictive Values vs. the Standard of Reference

Some interesting examples of the attempt to define the accuracy of a diagnostic technique came from the literature on TMJ imaging. Indeed, the technical quality of the main imaging techniques, such as magnetic resonance imaging (MRI) and computerized tomography (CT) has progressively improved over the years, to the point that there are well-defined standards for the diagnosis of soft tissues (e.g., disc position abnormalities, synovial fluid) with MRI and for hard tissues (e.g., bone structures) with CT. For instance, the diagnosis of joint effusion is based upon the clinical evidence of swelling around the TMJ area and/or pain in the TMJ area during function and/or lateral palpation, but several studies promoted the need for imaging-based diagnostic techniques (Larheim et al. 2001; Emshoff et al. 2002). The standard of reference is surely represented by MRI, which can provide information about effusion and inflammatory changes in the TMJ (Rudisch et al. 2001). Due to the high costs of MRI, some authors focused their interest on US (for a review, see Manfredini and Guarda-Nardini 2009).

US is currently applied to many areas of the musculoskeletal system, finding a wide employ for the evaluation of joint effusion in diarthrodial joints, like the shoulder and the knee. Regarding the study of the TMJ, US has been suggested to be quite accurate to detect disc position abnormalities (Emshoff et al. 1997). An interesting early investigation aimed to assess the accuracy of US in the evaluation of effusion of the TMJ compared with MRI findings, which were considered as the gold standard (Tognini et al. 2003). The following sections on the description of the study design and report of main findings in the case of an investigation about diagnostic accuracy of an imaging technique are thus based on an edited, arranged, and commented version of the manuscript Tognini et al. 2003.

Description of Study Sample and Design The study group consisted of 44 patients who sought treatment for TMD. After a standard clinical examination, participants were scheduled on the basis of the presence of one or more of the following signs and symptoms (at least in one joint): TMJ pain, joint sounds, restricted, or deviated jaw function. Importantly, subjects with muscular disorders were not included in this study. The TMJs were evaluated in order to detect the presence of effusion by means of US and MRI. The two examinations were conducted by two blinded operators within no more than 2 weeks of each other. During that period the patients did not receive any kind of treatment. These features of the study sample and design were important to limit at best the possibility that diagnostic accuracy of the US was influenced by the operators' skill and/or by time-related changes in the TMJ status.

As in the case of experimental studies on bruxism, imaging studies must have a dedicated section for important technical features of the instruments and devices that were adopted in the investigation. In the specific case of MRI studies, all technical details and diagnostic criteria should be carefully presented to ease reproducibility of findings. Usually, minimal technical requisites provide that MRI with a 1.5 T with a bilateral circular (8 cm diameter) surface coil for both right and left TMJs study is used. The investigation protocol provided for a first axial scan "scout" from that have been established seven sagittal–oblique slices in lateral–medial direction and coronal sections deviated obliquely in posteroanterior direction. Sequential Gradient Echo T1 (TR=340 ms, TE=16 ms, FOV=15 cm, slice thickness=3 mm, matrix 256×192, interslice gap=0.5 mm) and Fast Stiir T2-weighted (TR=3500 ms, TE=27 ms, FOV=15 cm, slice thickness=3.5 mm, matrix 256×160, interslice gap=0.5 mm). Criteria for the diagnosis of joint effusion were easy-to-understand, since effusion was established by identifying an area or thin lines of high signal intensity inside the joint space (no effusion=no area or thin lines of hyperintensity).

The same details should be provided for the ultrasonographic examination, providing that all TMJs were evaluated by means of an US conducted by a blinded observer in the same day of the clinical assessment. In particular, given the relatively lower diffusion of the TMJ US with respect than MRI, a more thorough description of the technique may be useful for the non-accustomed readers' convenience. An 8–15 MHz linear probe was used. A 1 cm spacer was placed between the skin and the probe. A static and dynamic examination was conducted on both TMJs, performing sagittal oblique scans along longitudinal axis and axial scans along transversal axis of mandibular condyle. The articular capsule was shown as an hyperechoic line running parallel to the surface of the mandibular condyle and its width was measured as the distance between that line and condylar latero-superior surface with the subject in the closed-mouth position. The articular disc appeared as an hyperechoic line with a subtle hypoechoic halo, positioned above condylar hyperechoic line. Condylar latero-superior surface was evident with oblique sagittal scan as a hyperechoic line, whose irregularities suggested the possible presence of erosions or osseous remodeling. Ultrasonographic parameters to make a diagnosis of joint effusion were the following:

The presence of joint effusion was diagnosed as follows:

- articular capsule width of 3 or more mm
- hypoechoic area within the articular space

Importantly, the rationale for using the 3 mm value as the cutoff value was based on findings of a preliminary investigation showing that it is the best threshold to discriminate between clinically relevant effusion and asymptomatic joints (Manfredini et al. 2003a).

Ultrasonographic findings of effusion were compared with MRI ones. Sensitivity, specificity, predictive positive values (PPV), and predictive negative values (NPV) were calculated. The agreement between the two diagnostic methods was then evaluated by means of Cohen's K test.

Description of Main Findings In this kind of investigation, results should be reported according to a basic strategy following the main points listed below:

1. Findings of the gold-standard examination (i.e., MRI);
2. Findings of the examination for which diagnostic accuracy should be tested (i.e., US);
3. Findings of the agreement assessments between the two techniques.

Thus, the number/percentage of joints with intra-articular effusion was reported for both techniques, and details of the comparison assessment were then described. The cross-tabulation of findings in a 2×2 table is the most suitable strategy to visualize and to assess the agreement between the two techniques (MRI vs. US) by using simple formulae, where:

- Accuracy is the percentage of correct US diagnoses (i.e., true US negative + true US positive findings/total observations);
- Sensitivity is assessed as true US positive findings/total number of MRI positive findings;
- Specificity is assessed as true US negative findings/total number of MRI negative findings;
- PPV is assessed as true US positive findings/total number of US positive findings;
- NPV is assessed as true negative US negative findings/total number of US negative findings.

Table 3.2 Cross-tabulation of findings: diagnosis of TMJ effusion with MRI vs. US. (Data are based on the paper Tognini et al. 2003)

	MRI no effusion (n)	MRI effusion (n)
US no effusion (n)	36	10
US effusion (n)	11	31

In the above investigation on the comparison of US vs. MRI findings, the agreement between the two diagnostic techniques was high for both joints with no effusion (only 10 of 46 were false negative) and joints with effusion (only 11 of 42 were false positive). Therefore, US showed a sensitivity of 75.6 % and a specificity of 76.5 %. The PPV and NPV were 73.8 % and 78.2 % respectively. US vs. MRI agreement for the diagnosis of TMJ effusion was good (pct. agreement 76.1 %; Cohen's $K=0.521$) (Table 3.2).

3.3 How to Assess Diagnostic Accuracy with Dichotomic Variables: Correlation Analysis between Findings of Two Different Techniques

Other interesting examples on how to compare the accuracy of a diagnostic device in the field of orofacial pain and TMD came from the literature on the various instrumental devices that over the years have been proposed as tools to measure TMJ and jaw muscles' dysfunction.

Statement of the Problem In the case of instrumental approaches to the assessment of TMJ dysfunction, it is well known that ethical issues are of major importance due to the costs associated with the adoption of such techniques as surface electromyography (sEMG) and postural platforms. Indeed, there are some clinicians who argue for using more technological devices in the diagnosis of TMD, but their treatment protocols seem to be associated with a very high risk for overtreatment and an unfavorable risk/cost to benefit ratio with respect to traditional conservative, clinically based diagnoses and interventions. In the clinical setting, instruments for making electromyographic (EMG) and kinesiographic (KG) recordings have been proposed as diagnostic aids for TMJ and jaw muscle disorders on the basis of their claimed usefulness to detect dysfunctions of the stomatognathic system. As in the case of the above US vs. MRI example, the most suitable strategy to avoid confusion and to ease the science transfer process is to perform diagnostic accuracy studies, in order to obtain findings that can be easily interpreted for their impact in the everyday clinical practice. Such a statement is mostly true if one considers the fact that parameters for physiology with the use of those instruments (i.e., KG, EMG) were not based on validation studies, and are drawn from the opinions of the users (Cooper 2004). No studies have been reported previously about the accuracy of KG recordings to detect TMJ disorders such as various forms of disc displacements and/or joint effusions. On this purpose, it must be borne in mind that MRI has to be assumed as the standard of reference for visualizing those signs and trying to correlate them with either clinical or other instrumental findings.

Considering these premises, an interesting example investigation is described below (Manfredini et al. 2012b). The main aim was to assess the correlation between magnetic resonance findings of TMJ disc displacement and effusion and some parameters drawn from KG recordings of jaw motion. In a similar investigation, which has important scientific, clinical, commercial, and ethical implications, it is important that (1) the authors have no conflicts of interests to avoid publication bias, and (2) the study findings are presented in terms of their confirmation or rebuttal of a null hypothesis under testing. In that case, the null hypothesis was that no correlation exists between MRI and KG signs. The following sections on the description of the study design and report of main findings in the case of an investigation assessing the diagnostic accuracy in the case of dichotomic variables are thus based on an edited, arranged, and commented version of the manuscript Manfredini et al. 2012b.

Description of Study Sample and Design Participants to the study were selected among those subjects for whom the need to undergo magnetic resonance was clinically established in the attempt to get deeper into the assessment of internal derangements and/or differential diagnosis with other muscle or joint disorders. Those individuals underwent a KG recording in the same day in which the MRI was performed. Exclusion criteria were the presence of systemic diseases affecting joint and/or masticatory muscles that could have altered the TMJ status, such as fibromyalgia or other rheumatic diseases diagnosed according to the American College of Rheumatology criteria.

MRI was carried out with the same parameters as described above, and images were made with the subjects at both closed mouth and maximum opening mouth positions. As an important specification, it must be pointed out that the latter position was obtained by means of a wooden intermaxillary device at the same opening as measured clinically, in order to avoid possible bias due to a sub-maximal opening during the MRI examination.

Then, specific criteria taken from the mainstream literature were adopted to diagnose disc position abnormalities and presented in details: The articular disc was directly identified, in sagittal oblique T1-weighted images, as an area of hypointensity with a biconcave shape above the condylar structure, and its position has been categorized according to literature data (Orsini et al. 1999) as either (1) Superior (normal) disc position (N), (2) Disc displacement with reduction (DDR), (3) Disc displacement without reduction (DDNR).

Joint effusion has been identified in T2-weighted images, which were more suitable to depict joint fluid accumulation, as a large area of high signal intensity inside the joint space, in accordance with the hypothesis that mild to moderate amount of fluid can be detected in normal joints as well (Manfredini et al. 2003a, b).

A further step to be considered is the need for addressing possible observation bias. Thus, to avoid interpretation bias related with the different radiologists assessing the images, MRI were interpreted by two expert clinicians, who recorded the presence/absence of effusion and disc position abnormalities by consensus.

The same attention for the technical details should be put in describing the other instrumental recordings under investigation (i.e., KG recording with a commercially available device). An interesting feature of such an investigation was the adoption of an instrument for jaw KG recordings that is available on routine bases for clinicians throughout the world, and it was claimed by the manufacturer as being a valuable tool for the management of TMJ disorders. The adoption of that device was an appreciable strategy to ease the so-called science transfer process, which in most cases is limited by the adoption of ad hoc instruments in the research setting that are not available in the clinical setting. During all exams, which were performed with strict observance of the manufacturer's guidelines, the patient was seated on a wooden high-backed chair, with the trunk perpendicular to the floor and the head upright, in a position achieved by asking the patient to look ahead. Some strategies were also adopted to increase the internal validity of findings detected with the KG: All tasks were performed by the patients three times at 10-minute intervals and the average value of the three attempts was recorded, and all KG assessments were made by an investigator with expertise in the use of such devices and with continued education training at in-house courses organized by the manufacturer. For all participants, a series of parameters were recorded for statistical analysis, based on their purported relevancy as markers for disc displacement and effusion: (1) maximum lateral deviation, (2) maximum lateral deflection, (3) KG incisure. Specific figures were provided in the original manuscript to help readers visualize the above markers (Manfredini et al. 2012b).

For statistical purposes and comparison with MRI findings, all KG parameters were dichotomized into categorical (yes/no) variables: Deviations and deflections from the mid-sagittal plane were considered positive for values higher than 2.5 mm, while the presence of KG incisures was considered positive when more than one variation (sudden decrease–increase effect) in speed velocity occurred during jaw opening.

A binary single variable regression analysis was performed to assess the correlation between the MRI findings (per each side: DDR, DDNR, effusion) and the KG parameters (lateral deviation, lateral deflection, incisures). The same strategy as described for the multiple variable assessment of occlusal risk factors for bruxism was here adopted: In the case that more than one KG variables showed a p value of 0.10 or less with any MRI findings at the single variable regression analysis, they were managed as potential predictors of the specific MRI diagnosis and were then entered into a multiple regression analysis as independent variable(s) to describe predictive models for MRI diagnoses.

Description of Main Findings The sequence of findings described in the results section followed the same strategy as defined for the example investigation comparing MRI and US, with separate paragraphs reporting the MRI diagnoses and the KG findings. Then, results of the correlation analyses were presented.

In particular, the presence of MRI-depicted DDR was not related with any of the KG findings, with p values ranging from 0.062 to 0.999. KG findings were not found related with MRI-depicted DDNR (p values ranging from 0.063 to 0.999). Also, the presence of MRI-depicted joint effusion was not related with any of the KG findings, with p values ranging from 0.09 to 0.999. An example table reporting all correlation values is really useful to give readers an immediate appraisal of the poor correlation between KG and MRI findings (Table 3.3).

Table 3.3 Single variable regression analysis. Correlation of the KG findings with MRI diagnoses based on data provided in a recent study on the usefulness of jaw tracking devices in TMD patients (Manfredini et al. 2012b)

			KG findings					
			Deviation		Deflection		Incisure	
			Right	Left	Right	Left	Opening	Closing
MRI diagnoses	Disc displacement with reduction (DDR)	Right	.036	.239	.079	.285	.225	.117
		Left	.345	.180	.206	.156	.045	.231
	Disc displacement without reduction (DDNR)	Right	.230	.099	.265	.070	.080	.070
		Left	.145	.338	.126	.070	.080	.070
	Effusion	Right	.071	.005	.015	.034	.280	.178
		Left	.054	.321	.163	.055	.215	.055

No correlations between MRI and KG findings below the $p = 0.10$ level emerged from the single variable regression analysis. So, multiple regression analysis was not performed. The clinical implications of such an investigation were enormous, since it allowed showing the poor usefulness of KG recordings in the clinical management of TMJ disorders due to their low diagnostic value for TMJ status.

3.4   How to Assess Diagnostic Accuracy with Continuous Variables: ROC Curve

The above-described investigation is an example of the poor clinical usefulness of jaw tracking recording devices in the orofacial pain clinics. Notwithstanding that negative evidence coming also from literature reviews summarizing the available knowledge (Manfredini et al. 2012a) claims for the usefulness of technological devices in the daily TMD practice are still diffused among clinical practitioners (Cooper 2004). Also, it seems that the quality of literature on the use of devices such as sEMG and jaw kinesiography (KG) is poor. In particular, the lack of normative values on which the discriminatory power between TMD patients and asymptomatic subjects should be based is a strong limitation for a definitive appraisal of their validity.

In view of these considerations, a possible strategy to try defining cutoff values discriminating between symptomatic and asymptomatic subjects is to use the raw data from continuous variables, such as EMG amplitude, and use Receiver Operating Characteristics (ROC) curve analysis to assess diagnostic accuracy. An example investigation (Manfredini et al. 2011) attempted to assess the diagnostic accuracy of commercially available sEMG and KG devices for myofascial pain of jaw muscles, which is supposed to be the main target for instruments aiming at detecting the muscle activity and the patterns of jaw motion for diagnostic purposes. The following sections on the description of the study design and report of main findings in the case of an investigation assessing the diagnostic accuracy in the case of comparison between two continuous variables by the use of ROC curve are thus based on an edited, arranged, and commented version of the manuscript Manfredini et al. 2011.

Description of Study Sample and Design Given the peculiar type of investigation, which needs to have maximum internal and external validity, an assessment of the needed sample size prior to the start of the study is a compelling requisite. The formula described in Chap. 1 was used to perform an a priori calculation of the needed sample size to detect clinically significant differences between a group of patients with myofascial pain of jaw muscles and a group of asymptomatics was based on data drawn from the literature, taking resting sEMG values as the main outcome parameter. A 50 % difference with respect to 2.5 µV, which was suggested to be the cutoff for abnormal sEMG values by a panel of expert sEMG users (Cooper 2004), was set as the difference to detect. Expected variance was set at 3 µV, on the basis of an estimated standard deviation comprised between 1.5 and 2.5 µV. This meant that a sample size of about 30 subjects per group was needed to achieve a 80 % statistical power (beta error set at 0.20) to detect a clinically significant difference with a 5 % probability to have a false positive error (alpha error set at 0.05).

Based on that calculation, the authors selected a group of 36 consecutive patients seeking for TMD treatment and receiving a Research Diagnostic Criteria for Temporomandibular Disorders (RDC/TMD) Axis I diagnosis of myofascial pain. An age- and sex-matched group of 36 TMD-free subjects with no RDC/TMD Axis I diagnoses recruited among the university staff and their closest friends. The latter control group was strictly composed by subjects who did not enter in any contact in the past with either the researchers involved in the investigations or the instruments under investigation to avoid potential bias due to preconceived ideas.

All study participants underwent an EMG and KG recording with a commercially available device, based on the recommendations of the manufacturers and according to the strategy described in the previous example study. The two examiners performing the sEMG and KG examinations were blinded to the participants' status, viz., being a patient or a control. For all participants, the following parameters were recorded and considered as outcome variables for group comparison: maximum mouth opening (in mm), maximum lateral deviations from the mid-sagittal plane during jaw opening (in mm), vertical free-way space (in mm), resting sEMG values for the four investigated muscles (in µV), sEMG values during maximum clenching on tooth and on cotton rolls (in µV), symmetry of muscle function, assessed as a raw ratio between the right and left muscle activity for masseter and temporalis muscles.

The average values in jaw range of motion and EMG activity were managed as continuous variables, and the existence of between-group differences were tested by the adoption of a T-test for independent samples. The level for statistical significance was set at $p < 0.05$, as usual.

A ROC curve analysis was performed to detect diagnostic accuracy (area under the curve), true positive rate (TPR [sensitivity]), and false positive rate (FPR [1-specificity]) of each parameter to discriminate between patients and controls. ROC curve analysis interpretation was based on the assumption that an area of 1 represents a perfect test, while an area of 0.5 represents a worthless test, viz., not superior to a coin toss. The closer the curve follows the left-hand border and then the top border of the ROC space, the more accurate the test; the TPR is high and the

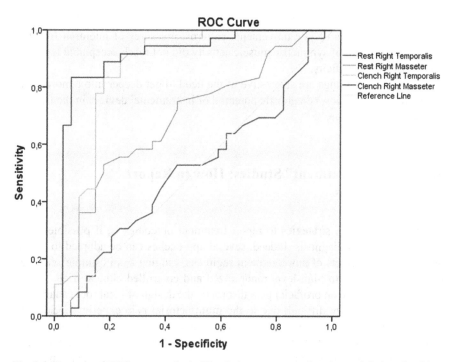

Fig. 3.1 Example of ROC curve analysis. Discriminatory power of resting and during clenching EMG activity of the right masseter and temporalis muscles to define subjects with myofascial pain of jaw muscles. The diagnostic accuracy is, on average, good for clenching EMG activity (the area under the ROC curve is above 70% of the maximum area) and very low for resting EMG activity, since the area under the curve is lower than 50% of the maximum area. (Data are arranged from Manfredini et al. 2011)

FPR is low. Statistically, a larger area under the curve means that it is identifying more true positives while minimizing the percentage of false positives (Metz 1978).

Description of Main Findings   Ranges of EMG data at rest in the four investigated muscles were similar between the two groups (i.e., 2.2–4.0 µV range in TMD patients and 2.9–3.8 µV range in TMD-free subjects). Differences between the two groups were not significant. EMG activity was markedly increased during clenching tasks in both groups, and TMD-free subjects achieved significantly higher levels of EMG activity for all the four investigated muscles, in line with the pain adaptation model postulating that injured muscles have a reduced motor recruitment. Measures of jaw range of motion and patterns of movements were similar in the two groups; also, the interarch freeway space in rest position did not differ between TMD and TMD-free subjects, and no between groups differences were detected as for the ratio between right and left muscle activity in patients and controls.

ROC curve analysis showed that fair to excellent accuracy (> 0.7) to discriminate between the two groups was achieved only with EMG parameters during clenching tasks (Fig. 3.1). Clenching tasks also showed acceptable levels of sensitivity (TPR, 77.8–91.7%) and specificity (76.7–86.7%). Resting EMG values had unacceptable levels of accuracy (0.28–0.48), sensitivity (43.5–52.2), and specificity (27.8–55.6). Also, KG recordings of jaw movements patterns, measures of interarch freeway space, and the ratio of symmetric muscle activity did not reach acceptable levels of sensitivity and specificity.

Again, these findings are suggestive of the need to get deeper into a more critical appraisal of the (low) diagnostic potential of instrumental devices in the field of orofacial pain practice.

3.5   Basic "Treatment" Studies: How to Report Case Series

The literature on the strategies to report treatment outcomes is, if possible, even vaster than that on diagnosis. Indeed, several approaches can be adopted to assess and discuss the effects of any treatment regimens, ranging from "simple" case reports or case series to high-level randomized and controlled clinical trials. In the case of the literature on orofacial pain disorders, the design of ideal root canal treatments (RCTs) is very difficult due to the multifactorial pain experience. So, it is not rare to find interesting findings also in some lower-quality papers, such as for example investigations reporting the outcome of some particular surgical interventions on the TMJ or treatment protocols providing viscosupplementation in patients with TMJ inflammatory–degenerative disorders.

The basic premise underlying those studies' rationale is that hyaluronic acid (HA) is a fundamental component for normal joints' lubrication effect, so that exogenous viscosupplementation was hypothesized to have a positive effect on TMJ disorders (Nitzan et al. 2004). Some early studies supported the efficacy of HA injections to treat TMJ internal derangements (Sato et al. 2001; Hepguler et al. 2002), but more recent evidence suggested that it may be effective in inflammatory–degenerative disorders as well, especially if combined with a thorough joint lavage (Guarda-Nardini et al. 2005, 2007). Such findings allowed extending the indications for TMJ HA injections to a wider population of TMD patients, especially in terms of age range, since inflammatory–degenerative disorders recognize a higher age of onset with respect to other forms of TMD (De Bont et al. 1997). Investigations on patients with TMJ osteoarthritis suggested that subjects of up to 80 years of age may benefit from a treatment protocol providing arthrocentesis plus HA injections, even if several aspects related with specific treatment effects have yet to be understood (Manfredini et al. 2010b). Among others, the effect of age on treatment effectiveness has never been assessed, so that it might be interesting to gather data on this particular issue.

In consideration of these premises, interesting data for discussion came from a study assessing the effect of treatment over time in different age groups of patients with inflammatory–degenerative disorders who underwent a cycle of five weekly arthrocenteses plus HA injections (Guarda-Nardini et al. 2012a). In this case, the null hypothesis was that treatment effectiveness did not change in relation with patients' age. The following sections on the description of the study design and report of main findings in the case of an investigation reporting treatment effectiveness by describing a case series are thus based on an edited, arranged, and commented version of the manuscript Guarda-Nardini et al. 2012a.

Description of Study Sample and Design The investigation had a retrospective design, and data were presented of 76 patients with a diagnosis of osteoarthritis according to the RDC/TMD Axis I Group IIIb (Dworkin and Leresche 1992) in the absence of both RDC/TMD muscle disorders (Group I diagnoses) and rheumatic diseases who underwent a cycle of five two-needle arthrocenteses with injections (one per week) of 1 ml HA and follow-up assessments after the end of the treatment at 1 month, 3 months, 6 months, and 1 year. The need to undergo the treatment protocol was based on the clinicians' judgment that patients may benefit from such an approach. All patients had a common history of pain lasting from more than 6 months, not improving, or improving minimally, with conservative physiotherapy or oral appliance therapy performed by their practitioners. The absence of authors' conflicts of interest (unsupported study, without any grants provided by the manufacturer) is a major strength of the study. Another important feature of the study, which is supposed to be read also by specialists outside the field of orofacial pain and TMD, is the thorough presentation of the criteria for diagnosing osteoarthritis according to the RDC/TMD guidelines, viz., presence of arthralgia, crepitus sounds, and radiological signs of TMJ bone structure abnormalities. The study also provided an interesting historical excursus to help readers comprehending the diagnostic criteria, by pointing out that the original 1992 RDC/TMD publication allowed plain tomography and panoramic radiographs to support the clinical diagnosis of osteoarthritis, while in the above investigation, as already discussed in some previous papers on TMD epidemiology performed in populations of Italians (Manfredini et al. 2010), plain radiographs were already available for some patients at the time of the first assessment. In some other patients, cone-beam CT was obtained to integrate the clinical diagnosis, despite this technique was not obviously available at the time of the early RDC/TMD guidelines.

The authors described carefully all the clinical parameters that were adopted as outcome measures. The basic instrument to measure pain reduction was the Visual Analogue Scale (VAS) from 0 to 10, with the extremes being "no pain" and "pain as bad as the patient ever experienced" respectively, as assessed by the same trained dental student at the time of the diagnosis (baseline), at each appointment during the treatment and at each appointment during the follow-up period. Also, measurements of jaw range of motion (i.e., maximum non-assisted and assisted mouth opening, left and right laterotrusion, protrusion [in mm], and functional limitation during usual jaw movements [0, absent; 1, slight; 2, moderate; 3, intense, 4, severe]) were provided.

Given the surgical and quite uncommon nature of the treatment approach, the injection technique adopted in the study was described in detail, in order to improve the clinical relevance of the findings.

The purpose of the statistical analysis consisted in assessing the effectiveness of serial injections of HA over time considering all the clinical parameters and taking also into account the effect of age. Patients were thus divided into three age groups based on tertiles of the variable age, in order to have three similar-size groups of patients under 45-years old, aged between 45 and 65 years, and over 65-years old. The responses (clinical parameters) were measured on the patients of each age group. All the outcome variables were managed as outcomes, while age was managed as a confounding factor based on the hypothesis that the real treatment effect could be affected by the age of patients if data were globally analyzed. Hence, a stratification of the sample with separate analyses was performed. A multivariate and multi-strata permutation test, based on the combination of dependent single variable tests, was applied. According to this testing procedure, for each univariate responses and for each age strata, a permutation test on ordering for repeated measures was performed, a first non-parametric combination of the results respect to the responses was applied, obtaining one partial test for each of the three age groups, and finally a second combination of the p values of these partial tests is performed giving a final global p value for the overall test (Pesarin 2001; Pesarin and Salmaso 2010). The initial univariate tests were also carried out using a combination based test, considering all the eight possible bipartitions of the dataset obtained pooling the first t times and the other $9-t$ times ($t=1,...,8$). Then for each bipartition, the mean values for the first t times and for the following $9-t$, a one-sided permutation test for dependent samples was performed to test the hypothesis of increasing or decreasing mean (depending on the considered symptom) and the univariate test was obtained combining the eight partial results related to the pooled samples. The combinations of the partial tests, at each level of combination (initial univariate test, within age group multivariate test and overall test), consisted in the application of the Tippett's combining function on the p values of the partial tests. Adjusted p values of the partial tests (according to the close testing method) are considered, to attribute the significance of the overall test to one or more specific partial tests. For all statistical procedures, significance level was set at $p<0.05$.

Description of Main Findings Results were described separately for each of the outcome parameters. Here, findings on the treatment-related reduction in pain levels will be described to example the strategy to report data on treatment outcome. A decreasing trend of the pain levels was observed in all the age groups but the shift for the younger patients, viz., those subjects aged less than 45 years, was less than the shift for the older ones. Notwithstanding that, the authors correctly pointed out that baseline differences between the groups were significant ($p<0.05$), with younger patients reporting less severe pain and thus being potentially less prone to report relevant improvement.

The global p value of the combined permutation test on ordering (with Tippett combination) was equal to 0.002 and, at significance level $\alpha=0.05$, it leads to the rejection of the null hypothesis of equality in distribution of the multivariate response for every age group over time in favor of the alternative, that is the symptoms improve over time. All the partial p values of the sub-tests related to the age groups, adjusted according to the close testing method for controlling the multiplicity, were significant: 0.009 (<45 years old), 0.001 (46–65 years old), and 0.001 (>65 years old), that is at significance level $\alpha=0.05$ there was a significant effect of the treatment on the symptoms within each age group and this is slightly stronger for patients >45 years old.

In summary, the adoption of such study design allowed the authors to show that for the younger age group the treatment had a significant effect only on the pain levels during chewing and on the subjective efficacy of treatment. For the other age groups the treatment effectiveness was evident on almost all the considered symptoms. An interesting interpretation by the authors was that in younger patients with TMJ inflammatory–degenerative disorders-like symptoms, the benefit of a treatment regimen with HA is lower than in older groups because of the fact that other disorders may be responsible for the symptoms.

3.6   How to Measure the Correlation of Treatment-Related Changes in Two Outcome Variables

In the above sections on TMD diagnosis, a couple of examples were provided on the use of instrumental devices, showing that their usefulness is much more lower than believed by some users. Also, it should be interesting to assess the potential employment of such techniques at the intra-individual level to monitor treatment. For instance, if one assumes that a reduction of one individual's pain level is the main marker for treatment effectiveness, it should be fundamental to evaluate the correlation of treatment-related pain changes with the modifications in KG parameters.

In an example investigation, the above described treatment protocol based on a cycle of five weekly arthrocenteses plus HA injections for patients with TMJ osteoarthritis, which was already suggested to be effective to provide pain relief and improve subjective chewing ability, underwent KG recordings of jaw movements at baseline and at the end of the treatment. Interestingly, the authors provided details of their working hypothesis and specify that the study protocol was designed to answer the clinical research question: Does a treatment-related change in pain levels and chewing ability coincide with a change in any KG parameters (Manfredini et al. 2013)? The following sections on the description of the study design and report of main findings in the case of an investigation reporting the correlation of treatment-related changes in two outcome variables are thus based on an edited, arranged, and commented version of the manuscript Manfredini et al. 2013.

Description of Study Sample and Design Participants to the study were recruited on the basis of the presence of monolateral TMJ osteoarthritis, as diagnosed according to the RDC/TMD Axis I Group IIIb, in the absence of rheumatic diseases. All patients had a common history of pain lasting from more than 6 months, not improving, or improving minimally, with conservative physiotherapy or oral appliance therapy performed by their practitioners. The presence of jaw muscle pain was not an exclusion criterion, proven that it was not the main source of patients' complains. The treatment protocol provided the same cycle of five arthrocentesis with injections (one per week) of 1 ml HA as described above, according to the technique described by Guarda-Nardini et al. (2008). To minimize operator-related bias, all interventions were performed by two trained operators with experience in the procedure. The study design provided that a clinical as well as a jaw kinesiography assessment were performed at baseline and at the end of the treatment. The clinical pain-related parameters adopted in the investigation were those usually adopted as markers of treatment effectiveness in previous investigations, and they were assessed by the same operator at the time of the diagnosis and at the end of the 5-week treatment. Again, to increase the internal validity of findings, the examiner who recorded the clinical parameters was blinded with respect to the findings of jaw kinesiography.

All study participants underwent two KG recordings, one at baseline and one at the end of treatment, performed according to the strategy described in the example in Sect. 3.3. Note that for speed-assessment tasks, the patient was asked to perform movements at the highest possible speed, and the maximum and average speed during jaw opening/closing movements were recorded. As usual, the investigator performing the KG recordings was blinded with respect to the clinical parameters. For all participants, the following parameters were recorded:

- maximum mouth opening (in mm);
- maximum lateral deviations from the mid-sagittal plane during jaw opening (in mm);
- maximum and average speed during jaw opening and jaw closing movements (in mm/s);
- maximum speed at the end of the closing movement (teeth-contact point) (in mm/s).

For statistical purposes, all clinical and KG parameters were managed as continuous variables. Three comparison strategies were adopted to assess the correlation between KG findings and the clinical parameters:

1. A single variable correlation analysis was performed at baseline to assess the correlation between the clinical parameters (i.e., pain levels and chewing ability) and the KG variables (i.e., maximum mouth opening, maximum lateral deviations from the mid-sagittal plane during jaw opening, maximum and average speed during jaw opening and jaw closing movements, maximum speed at the end of the closing movement).
2. Then, ANOVA test for repeated measures was performed to assess changes over time, viz., from baseline to end of the treatment, in all the study parameters. As a further step in the statistical analysis, a permutation test was performed to assess the correlation between changes over time in the clinical outcome parameters and changes over time in the KG outcome parameters. The permutation test was designed to test the null hypothesis that a treatment-related change in pain levels and chewing ability does not coincide with correlated changes in KG-recorded parameters. Specifically, the expected results were that if pain decreases and chewing ability improves, jaw movement speed and mouth opening increase.
3. Then, a single variable correlation analysis was again performed at the end of treatment to assess the correlation between the clinical and the KG variables parameters.

Description of Main Findings In the presentation of findings, the authors followed the same points that were described to present the statistical analysis.

Table 3.4 Significance of treatment-related changes over time in the clinical and KG recordings.It can be noticed that treatment of TMJ osteoarthritis is effective in reducing clinical impairment i.e., improvement in chewing ability and reduction in pain levels, but the KG parameters did not seem to change relevantly. (Data are summarized from the paper Manfredini et al. 2013)

Parameters	Average values	Significance of changes[*]
Chewing ability (0–10)	6.3±1.5 at baseline; 8.0±1.5 at end of treatment	0.005
Pain levels (0–10)	5.6±2.6 at baseline; 3.3±2.9 at end of treatment	0.002
Average jaw opening speed (mm/s)	68.7±42.9 at baseline; 71.8±40.5 at end of treatment	0.761
Average jaw closing speed (mm/s)	78.8±48.4 at baseline; 84.6±58.7 at end of treatment	0.658

[*] Significant at $p<0.01$

Table 3.5 Permutation test. Correlation levels between treatment-related changes in clinical and the main KG parameters. (Example data based on the paper Manfredini et al. 2013)

Outcome variables	Average jaw opening speed (mm/s)	Average jaw closing speed (mm/s)
Chewing ability	−0.218	0.199
Pain evels	−0.150	0.044

1. Single variable correlation analysis showed that chewing ability was not related to findings in any KG variables at baseline (p values ranging from 0.262 to 0.664). As for pain levels, correlations were found at baseline with average and maximum jaw opening speed and with maximum speed at teeth-contact point ($p<0.05$).
2. ANOVA for repeated measures showed that significant changes were described at the end of the treatment for both clinical variables, viz., chewing ability ($F=8.328$; $p=0.005$) and pain levels ($F=10.903$; $p=0.002$). No significant changes were described in any of the KG variables (Table 3.4). Interestingly, a good strategy in this kind of investigation should be to report findings of treatment-related changes at the individual level, in order to help readers visualizing the variability of findings and absence of correlation between treatment-related changes in clinical and KG parameters. A permutation test assessing the correlation of treatment-related changes in clinical and KG parameters showed that improvement in chewing ability was related with increases in mouth opening ($r=0.388$; $p<0.05$), and that both pain levels ($r=0.358$) and chewing ability ($r=0.366$) were related with changes in maximum left deviation during mouth opening ($p<0.05$). No correlations were shown between any of the other clinical and KG parameters (Table 3.5).
3. At the end of treatment, no correlations were found between the clinical variables and any of the KG parameters (p values ranging from 0.169 to 0.923).

Based on the above findings, the null hypothesis that changes in KG parameters for mouth opening and jaw movement speed were not related with changes in pain levels and chewing ability could not be rejected.

3.7 How to Compare Treatment Effectiveness of Two Therapies

Definitive information on the most suitable protocol as concerns the number of injections, the ideal HA molecular weight, and, more in general, on the most effective approach, viz., arthrocentesis alone or combined with drugs, is still to be gathered. Among these aspects, comparative trials on the effectiveness of HA drugs of different molecular weight may be useful to add information to the existing amount of knowledge on TMJ injections.

In view of these considerations, in line with the need to perform exploratory trials on the issue, comparative investigations were designed to answer specific research questions to try defining the best protocol for TMJ injections, such as: In patients with TMJ osteoarthritis who underwent a treatment protocol of five weekly arthrocenteses plus HA injection, does treatment effectiveness at 3 months depend on the use of different molecular weight HA? The null hypothesis of such investigation was that there are no differences between the protocols using the different molecular weight HAs. To test the hypothesis, the investigators compared treatment-related changes in some clinical outcome variables between patients receiving low vs. medium molecular weight HA (Guarda-Nardini et al. 2012). The following sections on the description of the study design and report of main findings in the case of an investigation comparing two treatments are thus based on an edited, arranged, and commented version of the manuscript Guarda-Nardini et al. 2012b.

Description of Study Sample and Design To address the research purpose, the investigators designed an exploratory randomized clinical trial. The study population was composed of consecutive patients with a RDC/TMD version 1.0 (Dworkin and Leresche 1992) diagnosis of osteoarthritis (Axis I Group IIIb) with joint pain lasting from more than 6 months, which were randomly assigned to one of the two study groups. Both groups of patients underwent five weekly single-needle arthrocenteses plus low-molecular weight HA and a 3-month follow-up period. This kind of investigation requires a description of the randomization strategy, such as an alternate allocation of patients into the two groups, which differed with respect to the different types of HA with which patients were treated, which was the same for all five sessions. As an important strategy for clinical trials, patients were instructed to have a 2-week wash out period before starting the treatment protocol and to not use medications on routine basis during the active treatment and follow-up periods (i.e., only paracetamol 500 mg was allowed in the immediate post-intervention phases).

To ascertain the needed sample size for the investigation, the primary outcome variable was treatment effectiveness based on the assessment of pain levels at chewing on a 10-point VAS scale with 0 being absence of pain and 10 being the worst pain ever. A priori power analysis based on literature data (Guarda-Nardini et al. 2008) and assuming a mean VAS value of $(6/10) \pm (3/10)$ in the main outcome variable, viz., pain at chewing, revealed that a 40-subject study design was needed to detect about a 40 % between groups difference in mean pain at chewing VAS values with a statistical power of 5 % for type I error, viz., false positive results, and 20 % for type II error, viz., false negative results.

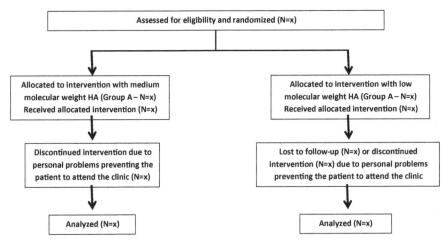

Fig. 3.2 Example flow diagram of the progress through the different phases of the clinical trial

For each patient, a number of secondary outcome parameters, viz., maximum pain at rest on a 10-point VAS scale with the same extreme points as the pain at chewing scale, subjective chewing efficiency (0–10 VAS scale with 0 being the worst efficiency ever and 10 the best efficiency ever), functional limitation, treatment tolerability, and perceived treatment effectiveness on a 5-point scale with 0 being the lowest and 4 the maximum values, jaw range of motion function in millimeters, were assessed. All variables were evaluated at baseline, at the end of treatment, and at a 3-month follow-up after the end of treatment. In the attempt to achieve a double-blind design, the patients were not told which of the two HA solutions was injected into their joint; they received a generic explanation of the potential benefit of administering arthrocentesis plus HA injections as well as an explanation that the specific intervention they were undergoing was indicated for their disease. For statistical purposes, VAS pain levels and jaw range of motion values were managed as continuous variables, while data on subjective efficacy and tolerability levels were managed as ordinal variables. For all variables, ANOVA for repeated measures was performed to assess the existence of significant within-group and between-group treatment effects. Adjustments for age and sex were performed to assess the influence of demographic features on treatment effectiveness.

Description of Main Findings A major feature of well-designed randomized clinical trials is the presentation of a flow-chart diagram describing the number of patients entering the study protocol, the allocation number in each study group, the number of patients completing the protocol, and the number and reasons for dropping out from the study (e.g., "*n* patients [*n* of the group A and *n* of the group B] failed to complete the treatment protocol [*n* subject] or to follow strictly the weekly appointments [*n* subjects] because of personal problems that prevented them to attend the clinic regularly") (Fig. 3.2). Also, the absence of significant between-group differences in sex and age as well as similar baseline levels in the outcome parameter are

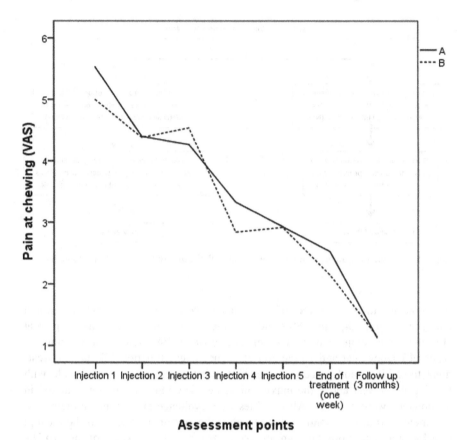

Assessment points

Fig. 3.3 Changes over time (x-axis) in pain at chewing VAS scores (y-axis) in the two study groups treated with different HAs. The figure shows that improvement over time was significant for both groups ($p < 0.001$). Between-group differences in changes over time were not significant ($p = 0.815$). (Data are edited from the manuscript Guarda-Nardini et al. 2012b)

important requisites to warrant that the comparison findings are not influenced by · demographic variables or baseline differences in any outcome variables.

In the example investigation, at the end of the follow-up period, both groups of patients improved in all the outcome variables. The effect of treatment was not different with regard to age and sex, thus being not influenced by the demographic features of the sample. No relevant adverse or side effects were observed in any patients, with the only minor exception of a transient anaesthesia of the temporal and zygomatic branches of the facial nerve area after an intervention in three patients. Between-group comparison of changes over time showed that differences were not significant neither in the primary outcome variables, viz., pain at chewing ($F = 0.056$; $p = 0.815$) (Fig. 3.3), nor in the other outcome variables (data not shown here [it must be noticed that the strategy of reporting outcome variables in a comparative clinical trial should be the same than Fig. 3.3]). Also, no between-group differences were shown for perceived treatment effectiveness and treatment tolerability.

The null hypothesis that there are no differences between the protocols using the different molecular weight HAs could not be rejected.

References

Al-Jundi MA, John MT, Setz JM, Szentperry A, Kuss O. Meta-analysis of treatment need for temporomandibular disorders in adult nonpatients. J Orofac Pain. 2008;22:97–107.

Cooper BC. Parameters of an optimal physiological state of the masticatory system: the results of a survey of practitioners using computerized measurement devices. Cranio. 2004;22:220–33.

De Bont LGM, Dijkgraaf LC, Stegenga B. Epidemiology and natural progression of articular temporomandibular disorders. Oral Surg Oral Med Oral Pathol Oral Radiol Endod. 1997;83:72.

Dworkin S, LeResche L. Research diagnostic criteria for temporomandibular disorders: review, criteria examinations and specifications, critique. J Craniomandib Disord Fac Oral Pain. 1992;6:301–55.

Emshoff R, Bertram S, Rudisch A, Gassner R. The diagnostic value of ultrasonography to determine the temporomandibular joint disk position. Oral Surg Oral Med Oral Pathol Oral Radiol Endod. 1997;84:688–96.

Emshoff R, Innerhofer K, Rudisch A, Bertram S. The biological concept of "internal derangement and ostearthrosis": a diagnostic approach in patients with temporomandibular joint pain? Oral Surg Oral Med Oral Pathol Oral Radiol Endod. 2002;93:39–44.

Goulet JP, Palla S. The path to diagnosis. In: Sessle BJ, Lavigne GJ, Lund JP, Dubner R, editors. Orofacial pain. From basic science to clinical management. 2nd ed. Chicago: Quintessence; 2008: p. 135–43.

Guarda-Nardini L, Masiero S, Marioni G. Conservative treatment of temporomandibular joint osteoarthrosis: intra-articular injection of hyaluronic acid. J Oral Rehabil. 2005;32:729.

Guarda-Nardini L, Stifano M, Brombin C, Salmaso L, Manfredini D. A one-year case series of arthrocentesis with hyaluronic acid injections for temporomandibular joint osteoarthritis. Oral Surg Oral Med Oral Pathol Oral Radiol Endod. 2007;103:e14.

Guarda-Nardini L, Manfredini D, Ferronato G. Arthrocentesis of the temporomandibular joint: a proposal for a single-needle technique. Oral Surg Oral Med Oral Pathol Oral Radiol Endod. 2008;106:483–6.

Guarda-Nardini L, Olivo M, Ferronato G, Salmaso L, Bonnini S, Manfredini D. Treatment effectiveness of arthrocentesis plus hyaluronic acid injections in different age groups of patients with temporomandibular joint osteoarthritis. J Oral Maxillofac Surg. 2012a;70:2048–56.

Guarda-Nardini L, Cadorin C, Frizziero A, Ferronato G, Manfredini D. Comparison of two hyaluronic acid drugs for the treatment of temporomandibular joint osteoarthritis. J Oral Maxillofac Surg. 2012b;70:2522–30.

Hepguler S, Akkoc YS, Pehlivan M, Ozturk C, Celebi G, Saracoglu A, Opzinar B. The efficacy of intra-articular hyaluronic acid in patients with reducing displaced disc of the temporomandibular joint. J Oral Rehabil. 2002;29:80.

Larheim T, Katzberg R, Westesson PL, Tallents R, Moss M. MR evidence of temporomandibular joint fluid and condyle marrow alterations: occurrence in asymptomatic volunteers and symptomatic patients. Int J Oral Maxillofac Surg. 2001;30:113–7.

Manfredini D. Introduction to TMD diagnosis. In: Manfredini D, editor. Current concepts on temporomandibular disorders. Berlin: Quintessence; 2010. p. 171–8.

Manfredini D, Guarda-Nardini L. Ultrasonography of the temporomandibular joint: a literature review. Int J Oral Maxillofac Surg. 2009;38:1229–36.

Manfredini D, Tognini F, Melchiorre D, Cantini E, Bosco M. The role of ultrasonography in the diagnosis of temporomandibular joint disc displacement and intra-articular effusion. Minerva Stomatol. 2003a;52:93–104.

Manfredini D, Tognini F, Zampa V, Bosco M. Predictive value of clinical findings for temporomandibular joint effusion. Oral Surg Oral Med Oral Pathol Oral Radiol Endod. 2003b;96:521–6.

Manfredini D, Piccotti F, Ferronato G, Guarda-Nardini L. Age peaks of different RDC/TMD diagnoses in a patient population. J Dent. 2010a;38:392–9.

Manfredini D, Piccotti F, Guarda-Nardini L. Hyaluronic acid in the treatment of TMJ disorders: a systematic review of the literature. Cranio. 2010b;28:166.

Manfredini D, Cocilovo F, Favero L, Ferronato G, Tonello S, Guarda-Nardini L. Surface electromyography of jaw muscles and kinesiographic recordings: diagnostic accuracy for myofascial pain. J Oral Rehabil. 2011;38:791–9.

Manfredini D, Castroflorio T, Perinetti G, Guarda-Nardini L. Dental occlusion, body posture, and temporomandibular disorders: where we are now and where we are heading for. J Oral Rehabil. 2012a;39:463–71.

Manfredini D, Favero L, Federzoni E, Cocilovo F, Guarda-Nardini L. Kinesiographic recordings of jaw movements are not accurate to detect magnetic resonance-diagnosed TMJ effusion and disc displacement: findings from a validation study. Oral Surg Oral Med Oral Pathol Oral Radiol Endod. 2012b;114:457–63.

Manfredini D, Favero L, Michieli M, Salmaso L, Cocilovo F, Guarda-Nardini L. Assessment of jaw kinesiography to monitor temporomandibular disorders: correlation of treatment-related kinesiographic and pain changes in patients undergoing TMJ injections. J Am Dent Assoc. 2013;144:397–405.

Metz CE. Basic principles of ROC analysis. Sem Nuc Med. 1978;8:283–98.

Nitzan DW, Kreiner B, Zeltser B. TMJ lubrification system: its effect on the joint function, dysfunction, and treatment approach. Compen Contin Educ Dent. 2004;25:437.

Orsini MG, Kuboki T, Terada S, Matsuka Y, Yatani H, Yamashita A. Clinical predictability of temporomandibular joint disk displacement. J Dent Res. 1999;78:650–60.

Pesarin F. Multivariate permutation tests with application in biostatistics. Chichester: Wiley; 2001.

Pesarin F, Salmaso L. Permutation tests for complex data. Theory, applications and software. Chichester: Wiley; 2010.

Rudisch A, Innerhofer K, Bertram S, Emshoff R. Magnetic resonance imaging of internal derangement and effusion in patients with unilateral temporomandibular joint pain. Oral Surg Oral Med Oral Pathol Oral Radiol Endod. 2001;92:566–71.

Sato S, Oguri S, Yamaguchi K, Kawamura H, Motegi K. Pumping injection of hyaluronic acid for patients with non-reducing disc displacement of the temporomandibular joint: two year follow-up. J Craniomaxillofac Surg. 2001;29:89.

Tognini F, Manfredini D, Melchiorre D, Zampa V, Bosco M. Ultrasonographic vs magnetic resonance imaging findings of temporomandibular joint effusion. Minerva Stomatol. 2003;52:365–72.

Chapter 4
Literature Reviews

Daniele Manfredini, Eleonora Carrozzo and Luca Guarda-Nardini

In the present chapter, examples of different strategies to summarize and discuss systematically all the available knowledge on different arguments related with temporomandibular disorders (TMD) are provided. In particular, the approaches to review the literature are discussed in detail by taking into consideration the bruxism literature: A first example review on the role of bruxism as a risk factor for dental implants is based on a PICO-like reading of the articles, and another example review on the epidemiology of bruxism. Also, a commentary on the factors to take into account when appraising findings from a meta-analysis is provided. As a general remark, it should be considered that several guidelines may be found in the medical literature on the best strategy to perform literature reviews on the different topics (e.g., epidemiology, diagnosis, treatment), so this chapter is not fully exhaustive of all the possible situations a researcher might be facing when attempting to summarize the available knowledge on a particular argument. On the other hand, there are some common suggestions to all the possible situations related to the search strategy, the inclusion criteria and the way to present findings as more neutrally and bias-free as possible. To those general rules is dedicated this chapter, which contains comments and suggestions that may help researchers searching for basic as well as more advanced advices.

D. Manfredini (✉) · E. Carrozzo · L. Guarda-Nardini
University of Padova, Padova, Italy
e-mail: daniele.manfredini@tin.it

E. Carrozzo
e-mail: carrozzo@gest.unipd.it

L. Guarda-Nardini
e-mail: luca.guarda@unipd.it

L. Salmaso et al., *Statistical Approaches to Orofacial Pain and Temporomandibular Disorders Research,* SpringerBriefs in Statistics, DOI 10.1007/978-1-4939-0876-9_4,
© The Author(s) 2014

4.1   The Need to Summarize the Available Knowledge on TMD

In recent years, much progress has been made as to the knowledge about TMD etiopathogenesis, diagnosis, and management. Findings that emerged from the literature have led leading researchers and academicians to claim the need for a less dentally based and more medically based approach to the assessment and management of TMD patients (Manfredini et al. 2012a). Notwithstanding the fact that this pathway is well appreciated within the research community, it must be pointed out that general dentists seem to be only partially aware of the ongoing paradigm shift involving the TMD literature. Indeed, it is not an easy task, once a new finding has been discovered, to diffuse it to the whole scientific community and then to the general practitioners.

At present, there are a large number of "scientific" journals and staying updated with the newest findings is often difficult even for those investigators who are involved in the process of scientific research and writing. It is not surprising to read position papers or attend lectures by academicians who cite only their own publications or studies that dated back to decades earlier. These publications or lectures are obviously less scientifically sound than other updated and more critical ones, and they are a frequent concern in the case of nonmainstream journals or events. Nonetheless, as pointed out by Greene in one of his papers, it still remains difficult for the general practitioners, the students, and even the colleagues from other medical fields, to actually comprehend who are the leading researchers and academicians (Greene 2006). Practitioners who subscribe to dental journals are a minority, and those who subscribe to scientific journals dealing mainly with TMD and orofacial pain are a small minority. Those people are not used to know the meanings of the words "impact factor" and are likely to be not able to use the Medline database.

Thus, the average general practitioner continues his/her post-degree education by attending some meetings and events and/or reading non-peer-reviewed dental journals. The main problems with this kind of continued education are the potential biases and influences due to the sponsorship of the events or journals. The diffusion of commercial information in the field of TMD practice has led to the widespread and irrational adoption of several technological instruments. This means that some further efforts should be made by leading academicians and researchers to diffuse their findings, and one of the best strategies for pursuing that issue is to perform high-level research summarizing all the available data on a certain argument.

The hierarchy of scientific evidence provides that publications are rated on the basis of the level and strength of information drawn from the studies. Meta-analyses and systematic reviews are the highest-ranked type of publication, since they provide a critical analysis of all the published papers on a particular argument (Durack 1978).

Despite there being several literature suggestions as for the criteria for the selection and inclusion of studies in a meta-analysis (Greenhalgh 1978), very few publications in the TMD field have been conducted in accordance to such criteria.

Moreover, most of them are not conclusive with respect to the key question they were intended to provide answers (e.g., role of an etiological factor; efficacy of a treatment or superiority over another one; accuracy of a diagnostic instrument), due to the poor quality of the studies that have been summarized.

Nonetheless, even if it must be pointed out the need for an increase in the number of high-quality studies, there are some strategies that can be suggested to perform literature reviews that give clinically interesting suggestions.

Based on these premises, examples of different strategies to summarize and discuss systematically all the available knowledge on different arguments related with TMD will be provided in the remaining section of this chapter.

4.2 How to Perform a Systematic Review of the Literature

In other sections of this book, some hints to bruxism studies have been already presented. The literature on bruxism is relatively "young," and it may provide nice examples on how to summarize findings on different topics. For instance, bruxism is a motor activity that is supposed to have the potential for causing damage to the stomatognathic structures as well as to be a risk factor for dental implants survival (Manfredini and Lobbezoo 2010). In spite of the increasing knowledge on its etiology, diagnosis, and management, evidence on the effects of bruxism as a cause of dental implants failure or complication is still lacking (Lobbezoo et al. 2006), and practical guidelines for the management of bruxism patients undergoing restorations on dental implants are based on expert opinions rather than on scientifically sound information (Manfredini et al. 2011).

So, there is a need to get deeper into the issue of the effects of bruxism on dental implants by performing systematic appraisals of the available literature on the argument.

Considering these premises, the below strategy is an example of a systematic review of the literature on the role of bruxism as a risk factor for the different complications on dental implants-supported rehabilitations, based on Manfredini et al. (2012b).

4.2.1 Description of Search Strategy and Literature Selection

A systematic review of the literature needs to follow some basic steps since from the early phases. In particular, a question to be answered through the review must be exposed (e.g., "Is bruxism a risk factor for dental implants?"), the criteria for including the studies in the review should be defined, and the medical database(s) (e.g., Medline; Embase; Scopus; Google Scholar) on which the search should be performed must be identified.

Then, all details on the search strategy should be presented. In the example review on bruxism and dental implants, which was lectured at the prestigious 20th Anniversary Congress of the European Association for Osteointegration (EAO) in Copenhagen (Manfredini D. Invited lecture. November 2012) and was then published in full version, the original search started some months before, on May 30, 2012. A systematic search in the National Library of Medicine's Medline Database was performed to identify all peer-reviewed papers in the English literature dealing with the bruxism–dental implants' complications relation according to the search strategy described below. The studies included for review were assessed independently by the authors on the basis of a structured reading of articles approach, which is also described in detail in the following sections.

A search with Medical Subjects Headings (MeSH) terms was used first. Such headings provide useful help to identify terms that can be useful as a starting point for a review. In the case of the bruxism and implants review, the two terms that were used to identify a list of potential papers to be included in the review were (1) Bruxism (defined as "A disorder characterized by grinding and clenching of the teeth", year introduced: 1965); and (2) Dental implants (defined as "Biocompatible materials placed into [endosseous] or onto [subperiosteal] the jawbone to support a crown, bridge, or artificial tooth, or to stabilize a diseased tooth", year introduced: 1990).

Additional details to the search strategy provided that the search was limited to papers in the English language and was then extended to the search words "bruxism" and "dental implants", according to the query: ("Dental implants" [MeSH terms] or "dental" [all fields] and "implants" [all fields] or "dental implants" [all fields] and "bruxism" [MeSH terms] or "bruxism" [all fields]). The search allowed identifying 77 citations, the abstracts of which were read to select articles to be retrieved in full text.

Despite the several potential strategies that can be adopted to define inclusion criteria, in that review the admittance was based on the type of study, viz., clinical studies on humans, assessing the role of bruxism, as diagnosed with any other diagnostic approach (i.e., clinical assessment, questionnaires, interviews, polysomnography, electromyography), as a risk factor for biological (i.e., implant failure, implant mobility, marginal bone loss) or mechanical (i.e., complications or failures of either prefabricated components or laboratory-fabricated suprastructures) complications on dental implants-supported rehabilitations by comparing the rate of such complications in subjects with and without bruxing behaviors.

Once those criteria are defined, a detailed report on the number of papers that were filtered at each step of the review is required. In most cases, it is also possible to present such report as part of the review's results. In the bruxism–dental implants review, after abstracts reading, 47 papers were excluded from further assessment because they were clearly not pertinent with the aim of this review and the exact number of papers excluded for the various reasons was reported, viz., the excluded papers were either review papers, articles expressing opinions or practical guidelines, papers in other languages than English, investigations on fracture analysis, finite element studies, single-patient case reports, or case series on selected patient populations. The remaining 30 papers were retrieved in full text and assessed for possible admittance in the review. Importantly, to warrant a good internal validity, the full texts were assessed independently by two of the authors and a consensus was reached in all cases to include/exclude papers from systematic assessment.

To search for other studies to be potentially included in the review, the Medline search was expanded: (1) to the articles related to the selected ones, based on PubMed suggestions; (2) to other keywords which were potentially identifying arguments related with bruxism (i.e., "dental occlusion", "risk factors") and which were combined with the term "dental implants" to retrieve other articles; and (3) to the reference lists of the full-text papers.

The methodological features of the selected papers were assessed according to a format which enabled a structured summary of the articles in relation to four main issues, viz., "P"—patients/problem/population, "I"—intervention, "C"—comparison, and "O"—outcome (PICO), for each of which specific questions were constructed in relation to the issue under review, viz., relationship between bruxism and implant failure.

The adoption of such PICO format means that, for each article, the study population ('P') was described in the light of the criteria for inclusion, the demographic features of the sample, and the sample size. The study design was described in the section reserved to questions on the study intervention ('I'), and information was gathered on all methodological features of the study, viz., longitudinal or cross-sectional-observational design, number of implants, type of surgical and prosthetic protocol, and follow-up period. The comparison criterion ('C') was based on the assessment of bruxism-related issues, by reporting the strategy to diagnose bruxism, to identify treatment success, and the related statistical approaches adopted by the authors to assess the role of bruxism as a risk factor for dental implants. The study outcome ('O') was evaluated in relation to the influence of bruxism to the outcomes of implant-supported rehabilitations.

All the above-described features of the included studies were put into tables, which also comprehend some critical considerations about the potential points of strength and weakness of the examined studies as well as the reviewers' response to the question "Is bruxism a risk factor for dental implants?" based on data of each single study. All the studies were assessed separately by two of the authors, and in cases of divergent assessments with regards to the assignment of strengths and weaknesses, consensus was reached by discussion. The element under discussion was deleted from the tables if consensus was not reached.

By adopting this detailed and controlled strategy for literature search and data extraction, the authors did their best to perform an unbiased systematic review providing findings with good levels of validity. Of course, some other approaches might have been possible, such as, for example, the adoption of a methodological quality assessment as a discriminant to include papers in the review.

4.2.2   Description of Main Results

After examination of the full-text articles retrieved from the first-step Medline search, the authors provided a nice example of how to report readers their study selection: 15 papers were excluded because they did not investigate for bruxism as a risk factor for dental implants ($N=10$), adopted bruxism as an exclusion criterion ($N=3$), or reported the outcomes of various rehabilitations in selected populations of bruxers ($N=2$). The remaining 15 papers were selected for inclusion in the review. Again, a detailed report of the successive search steps (i.e., Medline-related articles, other Medline keywords, and reference lists of the included papers) was provided, from which six papers were added to the original list of papers, thus accounting for a total of 21 papers to be discussed in the review. At a first glance, the findings of those papers as for the role of bruxism as a risk factor for dental implants were very inconclusive, with some papers supporting a positive association between bruxism and implant complications, some others supporting a negative association, and most studies providing uncertain results. Here, the authors did a good job in trying to grasp some interesting data for readers despite the foggy amount of investigations they were analyzing. Indeed, they decided to split the papers into those assessing biological complications ($N=14$) and those reporting mechanical complications ($N=7$).

Thanks to this split approach, some interesting suggestions could be drawn and presented in detailed tables, such as the template Table 4.1:

1. The 14 papers on biological complications accounted for a total of 3,447 implants, inserted in more than 1,000 patients. A large variability of criteria was also noticed as for the definition for implant success, ranging from literature-based criteria to measures of marginal bone loss, implant stability, or implant survival. In summary, bruxism was not related with implant failures in six papers, while results from the remaining eight studies did not allow drawing conclusions. Four of the papers with uncertain findings described a higher failure rate in bruxers, so identifying a trend toward a positive bruxism-implant failure relationship.
2. The seven papers on mechanical complications accounted for a total of 2,590 implants inserted in more than 700 patients. The mechanical complications that were investigated were variable, and included screw loosening, implant factures, and ceramics fractures. Multiple variable regression analysis to predict mechanical complications were performed in only two studies, which revealed contrasting findings of absence of relationship or positive relationship between bruxism and mechanical failures. The other five papers were either descriptive reports or investigations based on single variable analysis, yielding a positive relationship between bruxism and mechanical complications in three studies, absence of such relationship in one study, and uncertain conclusions in one other study.

Table 4.1 Example table of PICO-like structured reading of an article

Study's first author and year	Population	Intervention	Comparison	Outcome (bruxism-related)	Conclusions: is bruxism a risk factor?	Points of strength	Points of weakness
Author, year	45 patients (27F, 18M; m.a. 61.5 yrs.; a.r. 25–88)	297 implants 50 full-arch rehabilitations with immediate loading Follow-up 1–125.5 months	Bruxism (Unspecified criteria; 58 implants) Marginal bone loss—Implant success (Spiekermann and Jansen's criteria) Descriptive statistics	Higher failure rates in bruxers (29.3% implants [17/58] vs. 4.6% [11/239]	Uncertain	–	Risk factors not weighted Unclear criteria for bruxism diagnosis No patient-based data

m.a. mean age; *a.r.* age range

4.3   How to Perform a Quality Assessment
of the Literature

The literature on bruxism also provided interesting examples on how to assess the literature from a quality assessment viewpoint. A recent review was performed on the argument of bruxism prevalence in adults (Manfredini et al. 2013). An accurate estimation of bruxism prevalence is complicated by the amount of studies adopting different diagnostic strategies and investigating nonrepresentative populations. Therefore, estimates are commonly based on findings from a few large-scale epidemiological surveys, which suggested that self-reported tooth grinding during sleep has a prevalence of about 8% in general adult populations, with no gender differences and a decrease with age (Lavigne and Montplaisir 1994; Ohayon et al. 2001). On the contrary, little information is available on the prevalence of awake bruxism.

The literature on bruxism epidemiology was never reviewed systematically, so definite conclusions on the issue are lacking. Hence, the example below refers to the above-introduced systematic review of the literature dealing with the issue of bruxism prevalence in adult populations. Thus, the description of the search strategy, quality assessment, and main findings are arranged from Manfredini et al. (2013).

4.3.1   Description of Search Strategy and Literature Selection

Also in the case of this review, inclusion in the review was based on the type of study: original studies describing the prevalence of awake and/or sleep bruxism at the general population level by the adoption of questionnaires, clinical assessments, electromyographic (EMG), or polysomnographic (PSG) recordings. Studies performed on selected populations with comorbid medical conditions, such as for example TMD or psychiatric disorders, were excluded. All details of the search strategy were provided, with two authors performing the first step, and independently assessing the eligibility of papers for inclusion in the review. The other authors contributed to the expansion of the search strategy in the additional steps, and each of them also contributed with a handmade search in their own university library catalogue. The assessment of the studies' quality and data extraction from the selected studies were performed by the same two authors who performed the original search, and the strategies adopted for the quality assessment and for the data extraction were carefully checked by the other authors to minimize bias during the studies' review. In case of disagreement, decision was reached by consensus of the majority of authors.

The search strategy was similar to that described in the above example of the literature review on the role of bruxism as a risk factor for dental implants.

As a next step, the same strategy was adopted to identify papers in the Scopus and Google Scholar databases, and additional references were identified for inclusion in the review.

The final steps consisted of a search within the reference lists of the selected articles and a handmade search within relevant English-language peer-reviewed journals in dentistry, TMD, and orofacial pain field, within three journal Publishers' website search engines as well as within the authors' university library catalogues and personal collections. This final step provided additional full-text papers plus one abstract communication for inclusion in the review.

A total of 35 publications were found to be relevant to this systematic review's aim and were reviewed for qualitative assessment.

4.3.2 Description of Quality Assessment

The methodological quality of the included studies was assessed according to the checklist for the Methodological evaluation of Observational REsearch (MORE) (Shamliyan et al. 2011). The checklist contains six items to appraise the external validity, viz., the extent to which the results of a study can be generalized to the target population, and five items assessing the internal validity, viz., the extent to which the results of a study are correct for the subjects included in that study. Appraisal of external validity according to the MORE checklist encompasses evaluation of sampling strategies, sampling bias, estimate bias, exclusion rate from the analysis, address bias, and subject flow, while appraisal of internal validity provides an assessment of the source of measure, the definition of measure, validation of measures and reliability of the estimates, the definition of outcomes in subpopulations, and the reporting of prevalence.

A nice strategy to increase the quality of a review and the consistency and generalizability of findings is to include only those studies with an acceptable external validity were selected for further evaluation of internal validity and data extraction. The cutoff criteria for selection may be set as follows:

- Investigation should be performed on representative general populations (i.e. studies have to be excluded if performed on convenient, workplace, or health-care-recruited-non-general-population-based samples);
- Response/participation rate should be higher than 60 % of the target population;
- Study design should assess potential sampling bias, viz., it should ensure that all members of the reference population have a known chance of selection;
- Sampling strategy and response rate should be clearly reported.

Papers satisfying the above criteria for an acceptable external validity were presented in detail in the bruxism prevalence review as for their quality assessment and prevalence data. Also, some additional assumptions proper of the specialist literature on orofacial pain were made as to give homogeneity of the terms adopted in the different studies (Fig. 4.1).

Within these premises, for each of the included studies, the following data/information were recorded: size and demographic features of the sample (mean age (years) and gender distribution (female-to-male ratio)); type of diagnostic approach

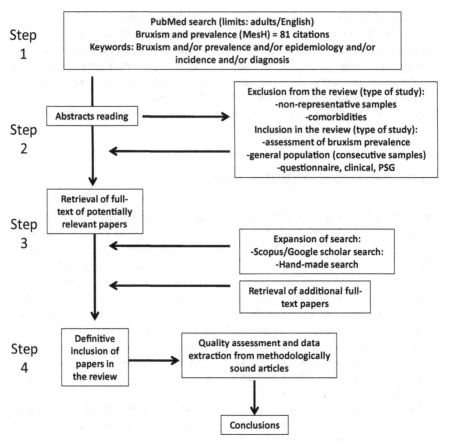

Fig. 4.1 Literature search strategy. Example of different steps and criteria for papers' selection in a recent review on bruxism prevalence in the adult population (Manfredini et al. 2013)

(questionnaire, clinical, EMG, and PSG); number of diagnostic items (N); presence of data analysis based on bruxism frequency, age, and sex comparison (yes/no); prevalence of bruxism (%), if available; prevalence of awake bruxism (%), if available; prevalence of sleep bruxism (%), if available; and gender- and age-related prevalence (%), if available.

4.3.3   Description of Main Results

In a review covering such a vast argument as the prevalence of a disease, quality assessment is fundamental to give homogeneity and consistency to the findings, since the reviewed papers covered a wide spectrum of populations of different age, gender, and ethnic background. Multiple studies were performed on subjects living in the USA, Sweden, Canada, Germany, UK, Turkey, Italy, Finland, and Japan. The sample size ranged from 100 to more than 13,000 subjects, with a very variable mean age of participants. A wide spectrum of gender distributions in the study populations was described. All studies except one relied on self-reported diagnoses alone, mainly based on one or two items. The prevalence of bruxism activities in both genders was assessed in 18 studies, an age group comparison was performed in 10 studies, and the frequency of bruxism activities (i.e., using terms like "sometimes", "seldom", "usually") was assessed in 6 studies.

Quality assessment showed that most studies had several methodological flaws. The external validity of findings was compromised by the very high percentage of papers with flaws in the sampling strategy (74.2% of papers had minor flaws and 17% major flaws, while an additional 5.7% had poor reporting of sampling strategy). Also, the exclusion rate of subjects from the prevalence analysis was not reported in any study, and there was a poor reporting of how sampling bias was addressed in the analysis in 91.4% of the studies. A specific table reporting the percentage of papers with the various shortcomings was needed as well as a report of the reviewed papers that did not satisfy the cutoff criteria adopted for an acceptable external validity and were thus excluded from data extraction and discussion.

The remaining papers, which were a strong minority (7 out of 35) were assessed for quality of internal validity, which was shown to be also a matter of concern due to the questionnaire-based approach to the diagnosis of bruxism. In particular, problems were identified with respect to the reliability and validation of the measurement (poorly reported in all studies), to the major and minor flaws related with the absence of an evaluation on bruxism severity and frequency, and to the minor flaws concerning the source of measure for the prevalence.

Based on that quality assessment, it was concluded that very few valid information could be drawn as for the prevalence of bruxism in the adults at general population level. For instance, given the heterogeneity of frequency criteria adopted to report bruxism as a whole and awake bruxism, consistent prevalence estimate could be drawn only for frequent sleep bruxism ($12.8 \pm 3.1\%$).

4.4   How to Assess and Comment Data From a Meta-Analysis

The highest-level reviews of the literature are those studies summarizing the findings from the available papers on a specific argument in a way that helps readers "catch" some statistical data derived from pooling the findings of each study and managing them as if they came from a single investigation. This approach is commonly referred to as meta-analysis.

While there are no doubts that methodologically sound meta-analyses are the best way to summarize numbers from the various studies, it must be pointed out that the literature search and inclusion in the review as well as data management cannot be performed only by professionals with expertise in statistics. Indeed, it is extremely important that professionals with a good specific know-how in the field of interest of the meta-analysis are involved throughout the whole meta-analytic process, in order to avoid bias in the study selection due the misinterpretation of clinical criteria for inclusion in the review. Also, in some occasions, despite being statistically sound, the conclusions from a meta-analysis are not clinically useful because they have low external validity.

The example below is based on a critical evidence-based commentary (Manfredini 2012) on a recent meta-analysis of the literature on the usefulness of temporomandibular joint (TMJ) ultrasonography (US) (Li et al. 2012).

The meta-analysis attempted to answer the question "How effective is ultrasonography in detecting disc displacement of the temporomandibular joint?" and was based on a literature search in the Medline, Embase, and the Chinese Biomedical Literature Databases with no language restrictions. Studies evaluating the diagnostic efficacy of US in detecting TMJ disc displacement; in participants with any symptoms or clinical signs related to TMD with use of MRI as the gold standard were included.

As a result, 15 studies (14 cohort studies and one case control) were included in the review, six of which studies had a low risk of bias, six studies an unclear risk, and three studies a high risk. Meta-regression indicated that the detected results were not influenced by the types of US, image dimensions, types of transducer, and ultrasonic image of the disc ($P = 0.05$). The Q* values (the point where sensitivity equals specificity on the summary reviewer operator characteristics curve) of US for the closed- and open-mouth positions were 0.79 and 0.91, respectively. The diagnostic efficacy of disc displacement with reduction had a sensitivity of 0.76, a specificity of 0.82, a positive likelihood ratio of 3.80, a negative likelihood ratio of 0.36, a diagnostic odds ratio of 10.95, an area under the curve of 0.83, and a Q* of 0.76. The diagnostic efficacy of disc displacement without reduction had a sensitivity of 0.79, a specificity of 0.91, a positive likelihood ratio of 80.5, a negative likelihood ratio of 0.25, diagnostic odds ratio of 36.80, an area under the curve of 0.97, and a Q* of 0.92.

The authors of the meta-analysis concluded that "The diagnostic efficacy of ultrasonography is acceptable and can be used as a rapid preliminary diagnostic method to exclude some clinical suspicions. However, positive ultrasonographic findings should be confirmed by magnetic resonance imaging. Also, the ability of ultrasonography to detect lateral and posterior displacements is still unclear." (Li et al. 2012).

An invited evidence-based commentary was asked by the editor of the journal "Evidence-Based Dentistry" to an author with specific clinical as well as clinical/research expertise in TMJ disorders, and some methodological problems with such a review were pointed out (Manfredini 2012).

It was commented that US of the TMJ has been the focus of an increasing number of researches over the last decade or so, and the review represents the first attempt to perform a meta-analysis of the available data on the diagnostic accuracy of US for TMJ disc displacement in comparison to magnetic resonance (MR). The reviewers commented that the intention of the authors was very laudable and the resulting paper is a useful statistical guide for readers willing to get deeper into the issue. The aim was clearly stated, the literature search comprehensive of three databases, and the data selection and extraction were performed meticulously. A flow diagram of the articles identified, screened after removal of duplicate studies, assessed for eligibility, included in qualitative synthesis, and included in the meta-analysis was provided. With respect to the most comprehensive systematic review on US of the TMJ conducted so far (Manfredini and Guarda-Nardini 2009), it seems that only one paper was missing from the reference list, based on the authors' inclusion criteria. Also, two additional papers were published after this review and were not included in the meta-analysis (Cakir-Ozkan et al. 2010; Bas et al. 2011). Findings from the meta-analysis suggested that the diagnostic accuracy of US for TMJ disc displacement is good to excellent both in closed- and open-mouth positions.

The expert reviewer concluded that, while these conclusions are statistically sound and the authors should be complimented for their methodological approach, it must be pointed out that they did not seem to take into account for the external validity of their findings (Palla and Farella 2009). The authors of the review failed to realize and discuss that six out of the eight studies included in the meta-analysis came from the same research group, and the other two studies, which described lower levels of diagnostic accuracy, came from another group (which was the one of the reviewer). Thus, redundancy problems cannot be excluded and cautionary statements on the need to perform additional investigations involving other research groups should have been recommended. This suggestion is supported by the newer findings not included in the review, describing accuracy values lower than the mean values reported in the meta-analysis.

So, as a general remark, it must be borne in mind that the management of statistical data by examiners without specific clinical expertise in the field of application of the meta-analysis may lead to potential statistically but not clinically sound conclusions.

Thus, along with some practice points (i.e., US may have promising applications to study TMJ disorders, it may be useful to replace MR in assessing the disc position for routine cases, and some other studies suggested that effusion may be also a target for US examinations), it was concluded that it is imperative that validation studies from more research groups are needed (Manfredini 2012).

All these observations suggested that, as a general remark, the conclusions of the literature reviews are strongly influenced by the study selection that, in turn, depend on the specific clinical expertise of the examiners managing the data. For this reason, it is not surprising that in such a peculiar field as the TMD and orofacial pain, some lower level, more narratively oriented, systematic reviews are still widely appreciated by the researchers belonging to the specific field of interest.

References

Bas B, Yılmaz N, Gökce E, Akan H. Diagnostic value of ultrasonography in temporomandibular disorders. J Oral Maxillofac Surg. 2011;69:1304–10.

Cakir-Ozkan N, Sarikaya B, Erkorkmaz U, Aktürk Y. Ultrasonographic evaluation of disc displacement of the temporomandibular joint compared with magnetic resonance imaging. J Oral Maxillofac Surg. 2010;68:1075–80.

Durack D. The weight of medical knowledge. New Engl J Med. 1978;278:773–5.

Greene CS. Science transfer in orofacial pain. In: Lund JP, Lavigne GJ, Dubner R, Sessle BJ, editors. Orofacial pain. From basic science to clinical management. Chicago: Quintessence Publishing; 2006. pp. 281–286.

Greenhalgh T. Papers that summarise other papers (systematic reviews and meta-analyses). Br Med J. 1997;315:672–5.

Lavigne GJ, Montplaisir JY. Restless leg syndrome and sleep bruxism: prevalence and associations among Canadians. Sleep. 1994;17:739–43.

Li C, Su N, Yang X, Yang X, Shi Z, Li L. Ultrasonography for detection of disc displacement of temporomandibular joint: a systematic review and meta-analysis. J Oral Maxillofac Surg. 2012 Mar 5;70(6):1300–9.

Lobbezoo F, Van Der Zaag J, Naeije M. Bruxism: its multiple causes and its effects on dental implants - an updated review. J Oral Rehabil. 2006;33:293–300.

Manfredini D, Bucci MB, Bucci Sabattini V, Lobbezoo F. Bruxism: overview of current knowledge and suggestions for dental implants planning. Cranio. 2011;29:304–12.

Manfredini D, Castroflorio T, Perinetti G, Guarda-Nardini L. Dental occlusion, body posture, and temporomandibular disorders: where we are now and where we are heading for. J Oral Rehabil. 2012a;39:463–71.

Manfredini D, Guarda-Nardini L. Ultrasonography of the temporomandibular joint: a literature review. Int J Oral Maxillofac Surg. 2009;38:1229–36.

Manfredini D, Lobbezoo F. Relationship between bruxism and temporomandibular disorders: a systematic review of literature from 1998 to 2008. Oral Surg Oral Med Oral Pathol Oral Radiol Endod. 2010;109:e26–50.

Manfredini D, Poggio CE, Lobbezoo F. Is bruxism a risk factor for dental implants? A systematic review of the literature. Clin Implant Dent Relat Res. 2012b Nov 13. doi:10.1111/cid.12015.

Manfredini D, Winocur E, Guarda-Nardini L, Paesani D, Lobbezoo F. Epidemiology of bruxism in adults. A systematic review of literature. J Orofac Pain. 2013;27:99–110.

Manfredini D. Ultrasonography has an acceptable diagnostic accuracy for temporomandibular disc displacement. Evid Based Dent. 2012;13:84–5.

Ohayon MM, Li KK, Guilleminault C. Risk factors for sleep bruxism in the general population. Chest. 2001;119:53–61.

Palla S, Farella M. External validity: a forgotten issue? J Orofac Pain. 2009;23:297–8.

Shamliyan TA, Kane RL, Ansari MT, Raman G, Berkman ND, Grant M, et al. Development quality criteria to evaluate nontherapeutic studies of incidence, prevalence, or risk factors of chronic diseases: pilot study of new checklists. J Clin Epidemiol. 2011;64:637–57.

Chapter 5
Nonparametric Combination Tests for Dentistry Applications

Rosa Arboretti, Eleonora Carrozzo and Luigi Salmaso

Considering the field of standard parametric or rank-based nonparametric methods, a large number of univariate problems may be effectively faced. Although in relatively mild conditions their permutation counterparts are generally asymptotically as good as the best parametric ones (Lehmann 2009), and for most sample sizes of practical interest, the relative lack of efficiency of permutation solutions may sometimes be compensated by the lack of approximation of parametric asymptotic counterparts. Let us also think of the situation where the responses are multivariate normal-distributed and there are too many nuisance parameters to estimate and remove, due to the fact that each estimate implies a reduction of the degrees of freedom in the overall analysis (note that "responses," "variables," "outcomes," and "end points" are often used synonymously); It is possible for the permutation solution to be more efficient than its parametric counterpart. Therefore, most parametric methods are based on several assumptions that rarely occur in real contexts, so that consequent inferences, when not improper, are necessarily approximated and their approximations are often difficult to assess. For instance, too often and without any justification, researchers assume multivariate normality, random sampling from a given population, homoscedasticity of responses also in the alternative, etc., so that it becomes possible to write down a likelihood function and to estimate a variance–covariance matrix. As a result, consequent inferences do not have real credibility.

Thus, the assumptions that parametric methods generally require are stringent and often quite unrealistic, unclear, and difficult to justify, and sometimes they are merely set on an ad hoc basis for specific inferential analyses. Thus, they appear to be mostly related to the availability of the methods one wishes to apply rather than with well-discussed necessities obtained from a rational analysis of reality, in

R. Arboretti (✉) · E. Carrozzo · L. Salmaso
University of Padova, Padova, Italy
e-mail: rosa.arboretti@unipd.it

E. Carrozzo
e-mail: carrozzo@gest.unipd.it

L. Salmaso
e-mail: salmaso@gest.unipd.it

L. Salmaso et al., *Statistical Approaches to Orofacial Pain and Temporomandibular Disorders Research*, SpringerBriefs in Statistics, DOI 10.1007/978-1-4939-0876-9_5, © The Author(s) 2014 accordance with the idea of modifying a problem so that a known method is applicable rather than that of modifying methods in order to properly deal with the problem. On the contrary, with nonparametric approaches, the assumptions are kept at a lower workable level, avoiding those which are difficult to justify or interpret, and possibly without excessive loss of inferential efficiency. Thus, they are based on more realistic foundations for statistical inference, and therefore, they are intrinsically robust and consequent inferences credible.

However, there are many complex multivariate problems (quite common in clinical trials, epidemiology, and biostatistics) which are difficult to solve outside the conditional framework and in particular outside the method of nonparametric combination (NPC) of dependent permutation tests.

We refer to Pesarin and Salmaso (2010) for an extended explanation of the theory presented in this chapter which represents a summary of some concepts suitable to understand how to apply multivariate permutation tests in particular to repeated measures designs, very much used in follow-up studies in dentistry applications.

5.1   Repeated Measures Problems and the Nonparametric Combination

In this section, we deal with observational or experimental situations where each subject is observed on a finite or at most a countable number of occasions, usually according to time or space. Thus, successive responses of one unit are dependent and may be viewed as obtained by a discrete or discretized stochastic process. This kind of problem is known as repeated measures design. With reference to each specific subject, repeated observations are also called the response profiles, and may be viewed as a multivariate variable.

Without loss of generality, we discuss general problems which can be referred to in terms of a one-way multivariate analysis of variance (MANOVA) layout for response profiles. Hence, we refer to testing problems for treatment effects when units are partitioned into C groups or samples, where C is given by the levels of a treatment and measurements are typically repeated k times on the same units. We want to test whether the observed profiles do or do not depend on treatment levels. It is presumed that responses may depend on time or space and that related effects are not of primary interest. From here onward, we refer to time occasions of observation, where time means any sequentially ordered entity including: space, lexicographic ordering, etc.

In the context of this chapter, repeated measurements, panel data, longitudinal data, response trajectories, and profiles are considered as synonyms. The proposed solutions essentially employ the method of NPC of dependent permutation tests, each obtained by a partial analysis on data observed on the same ordered occasion (time-to-time analysis). Hence, we assume that the permutation testing principle holds, i.e., in the null hypothesis, where treatment does not induce differences with respect to levels, we assume that the individual response profiles are exchangeable with respect to groups.

Formalizing, let us refer to a problem in which we have C groups of size $n_j \geq 2$, $j=1,\ldots,C$, with $n = \sum_j n_j$ and a univariate variable X is observed. Units belonging to the jth group are presumed to receive a treatment at the jth level. All units are observed at k fixed ordered occasions $\tau_1,\ldots,\tau_k$, where k is an integer. For simplicity, we refer to time occasions by using t to mean τ_t, $t=1,\ldots,k$. Hence, for each unit, we observe the discrete or discretized profile of a stochastic process, and profiles related to different units are assumed to be stochastically independent. Thus, within the hypothesis that treatment levels have no effect on response distributions, profiles are exchangeable with respect to groups.

5.2 Modeling Repeated Measurements

Let us consider a univariate stochastic time model with additive effects. Extensions of the proposed solution to multivariate response profiles are generally straightforward, by analogy with those given for the one-way MANOVA layout.

Let us refer to a two-way layout of univariate observations $X = \{X_{ji}(t), i = 1,\ldots,n_j, j = 1,\ldots,C, t = 1,\ldots,k\}$ or alternatively, when effects due to time are not of primary interest, to a one-way layout of profiles $X = \{X_{ji}, i = 1,\ldots,n_j, j = 1,\ldots,C\}$, where $X_{ji} = \{X_{ji}(t), t = 1,\ldots,k\}$ indicates the $j$ith observed profile.
Consider the general additive response model:

$$X_{ji}(t) = \mu + \eta_j(t) + \Delta_{ji}(t) + \sigma(\eta_j(t)) \cdot Z_{ji}(t)$$

$i = 1,\ldots,n_j, j = 1,\ldots,C, t = 1,\ldots,k$, where μ is a population constant coefficients $\eta_j(t)$ represent the *main treatment effects*, which may depend on time through any kind of function, but are independent of units; quantities $\Delta_{ji}(t)$ represent the so-called *individual effects*; and $\sigma(\eta_j(t))$ are time-varying scale coefficients which may depend, through monotonic functions, on main treatment effects η_j, provided that the resulting cumulative distribution functions (CDFs) are pairwise-ordered so that they do not cross each other, as in $X_j(t) \overset{d}{<} (\text{or} \overset{d}{>}) X_r(t)$, $t = 1,\ldots,k$, and $j \neq r = 1,\ldots,C$; $Z_{ji}(t)$ are generally non-Gaussian error terms distributed as a stationary stochastic process with null mean and unknown distribution P_Z (i.e., a generic white noise process). These error terms are assumed to be exchangeable with respect to units and treatment levels but, of course, not independent of time. When the $\Delta_{ji}(t)$ are stochastic, we assume that they have null mean values and distributions which may depend on main effects, units and treatment levels. Hence, random effects $\Delta_{ji}(t)$ are determinations of an unobservable stochastic process or, equivalently, of a k-dimensional variable $\Delta = \{\Delta(t)\ t = 1,\ldots,k\}$. In this context, we assume that $\Delta_j \sim \mathcal{D}_k\{0, \beta(\eta_j)\}$, where $\mathcal{D}_k$ is any unspecified distribution with null mean vector and unknown dispersion matrix β, indicating how unit effects vary with respect to main effects $\boldsymbol{\eta}_j = \{\eta_j(t), \ t = 1, \ldots, k\}$. Regarding the dispersion matrix $\boldsymbol{\beta}$, we assume that the resulting treatment effects are pairwise stochastically ordered, as in $\Delta_j(t) \overset{d}{<} (\text{or} \overset{d}{>}) \, \Delta_r(t), \ t = 1, \ldots, k$, and $j \neq r = 1, \ldots, C$. Moreover, we assume that the underlying bivariate stochastic processes $\{\Delta_{ji}(t), \ \sigma(\eta_j(t)) \cdot Z_{ji}(t), \ t = 1, \ldots, k\}$ of individual stochastic effects and error terms, in the null hypothesis, are exchangeable with respect to groups. This property is easily justified when subjects are randomized to treatments.

This setting is consistent with a general form of dependent random effects fitting a very large number of processes that are useful in most practical situations. In particular, it may interpret a number of the so-called growth processes. Of course, when $\beta = 0$ with probability 1 for all t, the resulting model has fixed effects. When dispersion matrices Σ and β have no known simple structure, the underlying model may not be identifiable and, thus, no parametric inference is possible. Also, when $k \geq n$, the problem cannot admit any parametric solution (see Chung and Fraser 1958 and Blair et al. 1994).

Among the many possible specifications of models for individual effects, one of these assumes that terms $\Delta_{ji}(t)$ behave according to an AR(1) process:

$$\Delta_{ji}(0) = 0; \Delta_{ji}(t) = \gamma(t) \cdot \Delta_{ji}(t-1) + \beta(\eta_j(t)) \cdot W_{ji}(t),$$

$i = 1, \ldots, n_j, \ j = 1, \ldots, C, \ t = 1, \ldots, k$, where $W_{ji}(t)$ represent random contributions interpreting deviates of individual behavior $\gamma(t)$ are autoregressive parameters which are assumed to be independent of treatment levels and units, but not time $\beta(\eta_j(t)), \ t = 1, \ldots, k$ are time-varying scale coefficients of autoregressive parameters, which may depend on the main effects. By assumption, the terms $W_{ji}(t)$ have null mean value, unspecified distributions, and are possibly time-dependent, so that they may behave as a stationary stochastic process.

A simplification of the previous model considers a regression-type form such as

$$\Delta_{ji}(t) = \gamma_j(t) + \beta(t) \cdot W_{ji}(t), i = 1, \ldots, n_j, \ j = 1, \ldots, C, t = 1, \ldots, k.$$

Of course, many other models of dependence errors might be taken into consideration, including situations where matrices Σ and β are both full.

The hypotheses we wish to test are

$$H_0 : \left\{ \mathbf{X}_1 \overset{d}{=} \ldots \overset{d}{=} \mathbf{X}_C \right\} = \left\{ X_1(t) \overset{d}{=} \ldots \overset{d}{=} X_C(t), \ t = 1, \ldots, k \right\}$$

against $H_1 : \left\{ \bigcup_t H_{0t} \text{ is not true} \right\}$.

The global null hypothesis can be written referring to the so-called time-to-time analysis, i.e., it can be seen as decomposed into k subhypotheses according to time

$$H_0 : \left\{ \bigcap_{t=1}^{k} \left[X_1(t) \overset{d}{=} \ldots \overset{d}{=} X_C(t) \right] \right\} = \left\{ \bigcap_{t=1}^{k} H_{0t} \right\} \text{ against } H_1 = \left\{ \bigcup_t H_{1t} \right\}. \text{ Note that } H_0 \text{ is}$$

true if and only if all the sub-hypotheses are jointly true and the alternative is true if only one of the k alternatives is true. By this decomposition, each subproblem is reduced to a one-way ANOVA, and from this point of view, the associated two-way ANOVA, in which effects due to time are not of interest, becomes equivalent to a one-way MANOVA.

Distributional assumptions imply that $X = X_1 \uplus \ldots \uplus X_C$ is a set of sufficient statistics for the problem in H_0. The permutation testing principle can be applied to observed time profiles because $H_0 = \{X_1 = \ldots = X_C\}$ implies that the observed profiles are exchangeable with respect to treatment levels.

Thus, in the given conditions, let us consider k partial tests, $T_t = \sum_j n_j \cdot (\bar{X}_j)^2$ where $\bar{X}_j = \sum_i X_{ji}(t)/n_j$, $t = 1, \ldots, k$, are appropriate for time-to-time subhypotheses H_{0t} against H_{1t}. In order to compute the k p-values we need the permutation distribution $(T_1^*, \ldots, T_k^*)$ under H_0 of $(T_1, \ldots, T_k)$. We estimate this distribution by permuting a number B of times the original profiles among the groups and computing at each permutation the statistic $T_t^{*b} = \sum_j n_j \cdot (\bar{X}_j^{*b})^2$, $\bar{X}_j^{*b} = \sum_i X_{ji}^*(t)/n_j$, $t = 1, \ldots, k$, $b = 1, \ldots, B$, where with the symbol "*," we mean that the statistics are computed on a permutation of data. On this null distribution, we can compute the p-values of the k partial tests by $\frac{\#(T_t^* \geq T_t)}{B}$, i.e., the proportion of times in which we observe a value of T_t^* greater than the value T_t observed on original data. Now, we can achieve a global complete solution for H_0 against H_1, by combining all these partial tests. Of course, due to the complexity of the problem and to the unknown k-dimensional distribution of $(T_1, \ldots, T_k)$ (see Crowder and Hand 1990; Diggle et al. 2002), we are generally unable to evaluate all dependence relations among partial tests directly from X. Therefore, this combination should be nonparametric and may be obtained through any combining function $\psi \in C$, where C is a class of combining functions that are characterized by the following property: (1) a combining function must be nonincreasing in each argument: $\psi(\ldots, \lambda_t, \ldots) \geq \psi(\ldots, \lambda_t', \ldots)$ if $\lambda_t < \lambda_t'$, where $\lambda_t, t \in \{1, \ldots, k\}$ is the p-value related to the t-th partial hypothesis. Also, it is generally desirable that is symmetric, i.e., invariant with respect to rearrangements of the entry arguments $\psi(\lambda_{u_1}, \ldots, \lambda_{u_k})$, where $(u_1, \ldots, u_k)$ is any permutation of $(1, \ldots, k)$; (2) every combining function must attain its supremum value $\bar{\psi}$, possibly not finite, even when only one argument attains zero $\psi(\ldots, \lambda_t, \ldots) \to \bar{\psi}$ if $\lambda_t \to 0, t \in \{1, \ldots, k\}$; c) $\forall \alpha > 0$, the critical value T_α'' of every ψ is assumed to be finite and strictly smaller than $\bar{\psi}: T_\alpha'' < \bar{\psi}$. Some practical examples of combining function are:

- Fisher omnibus combining function based on the statistic $\psi_F = -2\sum_{t=1}^k \log(\lambda_t)$;
- Liptak combining function based on the statistic $\psi_L = \sum_{t=1}^k \Phi^{-1}(1 - \lambda_t)$, where Φ is the standard normal CDF;
- Tippett combination function based on the statistic $\psi_T = \max_{1 \leq t \leq k}(1 - \lambda_t)$.

Of course, when the underlying model is not identifiable, and so some or all of the coefficients cannot be estimated, this NPC becomes unavoidable. Moreover, when all observations come from only one type of variable (continuous, discrete, nominal, and ordered categorical) and thus, partial tests are homogeneous, a direct combination of standardized partial tests, such as $T_t^* = \sum_j n_j \cdot \bar{X}_j^*(t) - \bar{X}_\bullet(t)^2 / \sum_{ji} X_{ji}^*(t) - \bar{X}_j^*(t)^2$, may be appropriate especially when k is large. This may not be the case when observations are on variables of different types, e.g., some continuous and others categorical.

5.3 Analysis of Case–Control Designs

Let us consider a particular case of the problem in previous section. Suppose to have $C=2$ groups and, for instance, we are interested in testing whether the first process is stochastically dominated by the second: $\{X_1(t) \overset{d}{<} X_2(t), \ t=1,\dots,k\}$. This kind of problem is known as two-sample dominance problem. In such a case, referring to models with stochastic coefficients, we want to test the following hypothesis:

$$H_0 : \left\{ \bigcap_{t=1}^{k} [X_1(t) \overset{d}{=} X_2(t)] \right\} = \left\{ \bigcap_{t=1}^{k} [\eta_1(t) = \eta_2(t)] \right\} = \left\{ \bigcap_{t=1}^{k} H_{0t} \right\}$$

against $H_1 : \left\{ \bigcup_t [X_1(t) \overset{d}{<} X_2(t)] \right\} = \left\{ \bigcup_t [\eta_1(t) < \eta_2(t)] \right\} = \left\{ \bigcup_t H_{1t} \right\}$, where $\eta_j(t), j = 1, 2$ represent the main treatment effects, and may depend on time. Note that the stochastic dominance problem is represented by a suitable decomposition of hypotheses. Observe that the alternative is now broken down into k one-sided (restricted) sub-alternatives. Hence, for each sub hypothesis, a one-tailed partial test for comparison of two locations should be considered.

The overall solution for this is now straightforward because according to the permutation principle, the exchangeability of individual profiles with respect to treatment levels is assumed in H_0. A set of permutation partial test statistics might be $\{T_t^* = \bar{X}_2^*(t), \ t=1,\dots,k\}$. Thus, we are able to estimate the distribution of $(T_1,\dots,T_k)$ so that we can compute the related partial p-values. These partial tests are marginally unbiased, exact, significant for large values, and consistent. Consequently, we can obtain the overall solution by NPC of partial tests.

5.4 Testing for Repeated Measurements with Missing Data

Consider a problem with repeated measures, where data are grouping into $C > 2$ groups and some of the data are missing. We want test the hypothesis if the profiles depend on treatment level.

Assuming that in the null hypothesis, both observed and missing data are exchangeable with respect to groups associated with treatment levels, such multivariate testing problems are solvable by the NPC of dependent permutation tests. Thus consider the hypotheses broken down into a set of subhypotheses, and related partial tests are assumed to be marginally unbiased, significant for large values and consistent. In this section, this NPC solution is also compared with two different parametric approaches to the problem of missing values: Hotelling's T^2 with deletion of units with at least one missing datum, and Hotelling's T^2 with data imputation by the EM algorithm (Dempster et al. 1977; Little and Rubin 1987). First of all, in this section we define two different situations: the first in which data are missing completely at random (MCAR) and the second in which data are missing not at random (MNAR).

Although some solutions presented in this chapter are exact, the most important of them are approximate because the permutation distributions of the test statistics concerned are not exactly invariant with respect to permutations of missing data, as we shall see. However, the approximations are quite accurate in all situations, provided that the number of effective data in all data permutations is not too small. To this end, we may remove from the permutation sample space, associated with the whole data set, all data permutations in which the actual sample sizes of really observed data are not sufficient for approximations. We must establish a kind of restriction on the permutation space, provided that this restriction does not imply biased effects on inferential conclusions.

In all kinds of problems, missing data are usually assumed to originate from an underlying random process, which may or may not be related to the observation process. Thus, within a parametric approach, in order to make valid inferences in the presence of missing data, this process must in general be properly specified. But, when we assume that the probability of a datum being missing does not depend on its unobserved value, so that the missing data are missing at random, then we may ignore this process and so need not specify it.

5.4.1 Data Missing Completely at Random

Let θ be the parameter regulating the distribution of the observable variable and let ϕ denote the missing data process; thus, the vector (θ, ϕ) identifies the whole probability distribution of observed data within a family P of non-degenerate distributions. The ignorability of the missing data process depends on the method of inference and on three conditions which the data-generating process must satisfy.

According to Donald Rubin: "The missing data are *missing at random* (MAR) if for each possible value of the parameter ϕ, the conditional probability of the observed pattern of missing data given the missing data and the value of the observed data, is the same for all possible values of the missing data. The observed data are *observed at random* (OAR) if for each possible value of the missing data and the parameter ϕ, the conditional probability of the observed pattern of missing data given the missing data and the observed data, is the same for all possible values of the observed data. The parameter ϕ is distinct from θ if there are no *a priori* ties, via parametric space restrictions or prior distributions, between ϕ and θ."

If the missing data are MAR and the observed data are OAR, the missing data are *missing completely at random* (MCAR). In this case, missingness does not depend on observed or unobserved values, and observed values may be considered as a random subsample of the complete data set. In these situations, therefore, it is appropriate to ignore the process that causes missing data when making inferences on θ.

5.4.2   Data Missing Not at Random

Let us think about sample surveys where it is very common to observe missing responses. These are situations in which circumstances behind nonresponses are varied and complex. Thus, the missing data might be missing not at random (MNAR). In order to make valid parametric inferences, the missing data process must be properly specified. Typically, in experimental situations this occurs when the treatment acts on the missing mechanism either on the missingness of a datum or on its observability. In general, it is very unlikely that a single model may correctly reflect all the implications of nonresponses in all instances. Thus, the analysis of MNAR missing data is much more complicated than that of MCAR data because inferences must be made by taking into consideration the data set as a whole and by specifying a proper model for each specific situation. In any case, the specification of a model which correctly represents the missing data process seems the only way to eliminate the inferential bias caused by nonresponses in a parametric framework.

In the literature, various models have been proposed, most of which concern cases in which nonresponses are confined to a single variable.

Let us present the permutation solution, considering a one-way MANOVA layout. Thus, the hypothesis to be tested is whether there is equality between $C \geq 2$, V-dimensional distributions. In order to do this, consider C groups of exchangeable V-dimensional responses $X_j = \{X_{ji} = (X_{hji}, h = 1, \ldots, V), i = 1, \ldots, n_j\}$, $j = 1, \ldots, C$, respectively with distribution function P_j, $X_{ji} \in R^V$, where $n = \sum_j n_j$ is the total sample size. Some of the data are supposed to be missing. Formalizing the null hypothesis is $H_0 : \{P_1 = \ldots = P_C = P\} = \{X_1 \overset{d}{=} \ldots \overset{d}{=} X_C\}$ against the alternative is $H_1 : \{H_0 \text{ is not true}\}$.

Assume that under the null hypothesis, data can be considered exchangeable with respect to C groups. This requirement concerns both observed and missing data. Let us assume that the model for treatment effects is such that resulting CDFs satisfy the pairwise dominance condition, so that locations of suitable transformations φ_h, $h = 1, \ldots, V$, of the data are useful for discrimination, where φ_h may be specific to the hth variable. This assumption leads us to consider sampling means of transformed data as proper indicators for treatment effects. The reason for this kind of statistical indicator, and consequently for this kind of assumption, is that in this situation we are able to derive an effective solution. Therefore, we assume that the analysis is based on the transformed data:

$$\mathbf{Y} = \{Y_{hji} = \varphi_h(X_{hji}), i = 1, \ldots, n_j, j = 1, \ldots, C, h = 1, \ldots, V\}.$$

Hence, consequent permutation partial tests should be based on proper functions of sampling totals $S_{hj}^* = \sum_{i \leq n_j} Y_{hji}^*$, $j = 1, \ldots, C$, $h = 1, \ldots, V$. Since for whatever reason

some of the data are missing, we must also consider the associated inclusion indicator, which represents the observed configuration in the data set:

$$O = \{O_{hji}, i = 1,\ldots,n_j, j = 1,\ldots,C, h = 1,\ldots,V\},$$

where $O_{hji} = 1$ if X_{hji} has been observed and collected, otherwise $O_{hji} = 0$.

Hence, we can write the whole set of observed data as the pair of associated
matrices (Y,O), and we can also define the actual sample size of the really observed
data in the jth group relative to the hth variable and the total actual sample size of
the really observed data relative to the hth variable, respectively by $v_{hj} = \sum_i O_{hji}$,
$j = 1,\ldots,C$, $h = 1,\ldots,V$ and $v_{h\bullet} = \sum_j v_{hj}$, $h = 1,\ldots,V$.

Note that, we may express the hypotheses of interest as

$$H_0 : \left\{ (\mathbf{Y}_1,\mathbf{O}_1) \overset{d}{=} \ldots \overset{d}{=} (\mathbf{Y}_C,\mathbf{O}_C) \right\}$$

against the alternative $H_1 : \{H_0$ is not true $\}$.

The complexity of this testing problem is such that it is very difficult to find a
single overall test statistic. *This kind of problem* may be tackled by means of the
NPC of a set of dependent permutation tests. To this end, we observe that the null
hypothesis may be equivalently written in the form

$$H_0 : \left\{ \bigcap_{h=1}^{V} [(Y_{h1},O_{h1}) \overset{d}{=} \ldots \overset{d}{=} (Y_{hC},O_{hC})] \right\} = \left\{ \bigcap_{h=1}^{V} H_{0h} \right\},$$

where, as usual, a suitable and meaningful breakdown of H_0 is emphasized. Hence,
the hypothesis H_0 against H_1 is broken down into V sub-hypotheses H_{0h} against
H_{1h}, $h = 1,\ldots,V$, in such a way that H_0 is true if all the H_{0h} are jointly true and H_1
is true if at least one among the H_{1h} is true, so that $H_1 = \bigcup_h H_{1h}$.

Thus, to test H_0 against H_1, we consider a V-dimensional vector of real-valued
test statistics $\mathbf{T} = \{T_1,\ldots,T_V\}$, the hth component of which is the univariate partial
test for the hth sub-hypothesis H_{0h} against H_{1h}. Without loss of generality, we
assume that partial tests are non-degenerate, marginally unbiased, consistent, and
significant for large values. Hence, the combined test is a function of V dependent partial tests. Of course, the combination must be nonparametric, particularly
with regard to the underlying dependence relation structure, because in this setting
only very rarely may the dependence structure among partial tests be effectively
analyzed.

Let us start considering a MNAR model for missing data, where it is assumed
that, in the alternative, the symbolic treatment may influence missingness. In fact,
the treatment may affect the distributions of both variables Y and of the inclusion
indicator O. Thus, in this setting, the null hypothesis have to take into consideration
the joint distributional equality of the missing data process in the C groups, giving
rise to O, and of response variables Y conditional on O, i.e.,

$$H_0 : \left\{ [\mathbf{O}_1 \overset{d}{=}...\overset{d}{=} \mathbf{O}_C] \cap [(\mathbf{Y}_1 \overset{d}{=}...\overset{d}{=} \mathbf{Y}_C)|\mathbf{O}] \right\}.$$

In the null hypothesis, the assumption of exchangeability of the n individual data vectors in (Y,O) with respect to the C groups is satisfied, because we assume that there is no difference in distribution for the multivariate inclusion indicator variables O_j, $j = 1,...,C$, and, conditionally on O, for actually observed variables $\mathbf{Y}$. As a consequence, it is not necessary to specify both the missing data process and the data distribution, provided that marginally unbiased permutation tests are available. In particular, it is not necessary to specify the dependence relation structure in $(\mathbf{Y},\mathbf{O})$ because it is nonparametrically processed. In this framework, the hypotheses may be broken down into the $2V$ sub-hypotheses

$$H_0 : \left\{ \left[\cap_h (O_{h1} \overset{d}{=}...\overset{d}{=} O_{hC}) \right] \cap \left[\cap_h (Y_{h1} \overset{d}{=}...\overset{d}{=} Y_{hC})|O \right] \right\}$$

$$= \left\{ H_0^{\mathbf{O}} \cap H_0^{\mathbf{Y}|\mathbf{O}} \right\} = \left\{ (\cap_h H_{0h}^{\mathbf{O}}) \cap (\cap_h H_{0h}^{\mathbf{Y}|\mathbf{O}}) \right\}$$

against

$$H_1 : \left\{ (\cap_h H_{1h}^{\mathbf{O}}) \cup (\cap_h H_{1h}^{\mathbf{Y}|\mathbf{O}}) \right\},$$

where $H_{0h}^{\mathbf{O}}$ indicates the equality in distribution among the C levels of the hth marginal component of the inclusion (missing) indicator process, and $H_{0h}^{\mathbf{Y}|\mathbf{O}}$ indicates the equality in distribution of the hth component of $\mathbf{Y}$, conditional on $\mathbf{O}$.

For each of the V sub-hypotheses $H_{0h}^{\mathbf{O}}$, a permutation test statistic such as Pearson's X^2, or other suitable tests for proper testing with binary categorical data, are generally appropriate (for testing with categorical variables, see Cressie and Read 1988; Agresti 2002). For each of the k sub-hypotheses $H_{0h}^{\mathbf{Y}|\mathbf{O}}$, $\mathbf{O}$ is fixed at its observed value, so that we may proceed conditionally.

Let us consider now the situation where missing data are MCAR. Note that in this setting, we assume that O does not provide any discriminative information about treatment effects. Thus, we can proceed according to Donald Rubin, i.e., conditionally with respect to the observed inclusion indicator O and ignore $H_0^{\mathbf{O}}$. The null hypothesis can be written as:

$$H_0 = H_0^{\mathbf{Y}|\mathbf{O}} : \left\{ \cap_h (Y_{h1} \overset{d}{=}...\overset{d}{=} Y_{hC})|\mathbf{O} \right\} = \left\{ \cap_h H_{0h}^{\mathbf{Y}|\mathbf{O}} \right\}$$

against

$$H_1 : \left\{ \bigcap_h H_{1h}^{Y|O} \right\}.$$

Of course, this problem is solved by NPC $\psi_Y \left(\lambda_1^{Y|O}, \ldots, \lambda_V^{Y|O} \right)$.

In order to deal with this problem using a permutation strategy, it is necessary to consider the role of permuted inclusion indicators $\mathbf{O}^* = \{ O_{hji}^*, \ i = 1, \ldots, n_j, \ j = 1, \ldots, C, \ h = 1, \ldots, V \}$, especially with respect to numbers of missing data, in all points of the permutation sample space $(\mathcal{Y}, \mathcal{O})_{/(\mathbf{Y}, \mathbf{O})}$ associated with the pair $(\mathbf{Y}, \mathbf{O})$.

Note that, units with missing data participate in the permutation mechanism as well as all other units, so that permutation actual sample sizes of really valid data for each component variable within each group, $v_{hj}^* = \Sigma_i O_{hji}^*, \ j = 1, \ldots, C, \ h = 1, \ldots, V$, vary according to the random attribution of unit vectors, and of relative missing data, to the C groups.

Thus, the key to a suitable solution is to use partial test statistics, the permutation distributions of which are at least approximately invariant with respect to the permutation of actual sample sizes of valid data. This is done in what follows. However, these tests are also presented in Pesarin and Salmaso (2010).

Let us first consider an MCAR model. Let T be a vector of partial test statistics, based on functions of sampling totals of valid data, and $Ft \,|\, (Y, O), \ t \in R^V$ its multivariate permutation distribution. The set of possible permuted inclusion indicators according to the random attribution of data to the C groups, say O^* of O, leads to a partition into suborbits on the whole permutation sample space $(Y, O)_{(\mathbf{Y}, \mathbf{O})}$, which are characterized by points which exhibit the same matrix of permutation actual sample sizes of valid data $\{ v_{hj}^*, \ j = 1, \ldots, C, \ h = 1, \ldots, V \}$.

This partition shows that the two points $(\mathbf{Y}_1^*, \mathbf{O}_1^*)$ and $(\mathbf{Y}_2^*, \mathbf{O}_2^*)$ lying on the same suborbit if the respective permutation actual sample sizes of valid data $v_{1hj}^* = \Sigma_i O_{1hji}^*$ and $v_{2hj}^* = \Sigma_i O_{2hji}^*$ are equal for every h and j, $h = 1, \ldots, V$, $j = 1, \ldots, C$.

Of course, if the permutation subdistributions of the whole matrix of sampling totals $\{ S_{hj}^* = \Sigma_i Y_{hji}^* \cdot O_{hji}^*, \ j = 1, \ldots, C, \ h = 1, \ldots, V \}$, where it is assumed that $O_{hji}^* = 0$ implies $Y_{hji}^* \cdot O_{hji}^* = 0$, are invariant with respect to the suborbits induced by $\mathbf{O}^*$, then we may evaluate $Ft \,|\, (Y, O)$ for instance by a simple CMC procedure, i.e., by ignoring the partition into induced suborbits.

Thus, the equality

$$F \left[\mathbf{t} \,|\, (\mathbf{Y}, \mathbf{O}) \right] = F \left[\mathbf{t} \,|\, (\mathbf{Y}, \mathbf{O}^*) \right]$$

is satisfied for every $t \in R^V$, for every specific permutation O^* of O, and for all data sets Y, due to the distributional invariance with respect to permuted inclusion indicators O^* of sampling totals S^*. Note that, for one-dimensional problems, this distributional invariance may become exact in MCAR models because, conditionally, we are allowed to ignore missingness by removing all unobserved units from the data set. But with V-dimensional ($V > 1$) problems, this distributional invariance can be satisfy exactly only for some particular conditions, or for very large sample sizes.

Moreover, when problems involve multivariate paired data, so that numbers of missing differences are permutationally invariant quantities, then related tests become exact. Therefore, in general, we must look for approximate solutions.

Let $V = \{V_{hj}, \; j = 1,\ldots,C, \; h = 1,\ldots,V\}$ be the $V \times C$ matrix of actual sample sizes of valid data in the observed inclusion indicator O, and consider test statistics based on permutation sampling totals of valid data $\{S_{hj}^* = \sum_i Y_{hji}^* \cdot O_{hji}^*, \; j = 1,\ldots,C,$ $h = 1,\ldots,V\}$. Note that, the following distributional equality

$$F[t \mid (Y,v)] = F[t \mid (Y,v^*)],$$

where $v^* = \{v_{hj}^*, j = 1,\ldots,C, h = 1,\ldots,V\}$ represents the $V \times C$ matrix of permutation of actual sample sizes of valid data associated with O^*, holds. In fact, the permutation distribution of the sampling total S_{hj}^*, conditional on the whole data set (Y,O) considered as a finite population, depends essentially on the number v_{hj}^* of summands. Hence, we have to find test statistics the permutation null subdistributions of which are invariant with respect to v^* and for all Y.

In general, in very few situations this condition is exactly satisfied, so that we must consider an approximate solution. Thus, we must look for statistics T whose means and variances are invariant with respect to the suborbits induced by O^* on permutation sample space $(Y,O)_{/(Y,O)}$. Let us suppose, without loss of generality, to have a univariate variable Y, so that we have only one test statistic T. Considering permutation tests based on univariate sampling totals of valid data, $S_j^* = \sum_i Y_{ji}^* \cdot O_{ji}^*$, $j = 1,\ldots,C$, the overall total $S = \sum_j S_j$, which is assumed to be a nonnull quantity, is permutationally invariant because in $(\mathcal{Y},\mathcal{O})_{/(Y,O)}$. Thus, the equation

$$S = \sum_{ji} Y_{ji} \cdot O_{ji} = \sum_j S_j^*$$

is always satisfied.

Let us now consider the two-sample case ($C=2$) and assume that the test statistic for $H_0^{Y|O}$ against $H_1^{Y|O}$ is a linear combination of S_1^* and S_2^*. Thus, the test is expressed in the form

$$T^*(a^*,b^* \mid v^*) = a^* \cdot S_1^* - b^* \cdot S_2^*,$$

where a^* and b^* are two coefficients which are independent of the actually observed data Y but which may be permutationally noninvariant. These coefficients must be determined assuming that, in the null hypothesis, the variance $\mathbb{V}[T^*(a^*,b^*) \mid v^*] = \zeta^2$ is constant, in the sense that it is independent of the permutation of actual sample sizes v_j^*, $j = 1,2$, and that the mean values should identically satisfy the condition $\mathbb{E}[T^*(a^*,b^*) \mid v^*] = 0$.

In accordance with the technique of without-replacement random sampling from $(\mathbf{Y}, \mathbf{O})$ which, due to conditioning, is assumed to play the role of a finite population, we can write the following set of equations:

- $v_1^* + v_2^* = v$,
- $S_1^* + S_2^* = S$,
- $\mathbb{E}(S_j^*) = S \cdot v_j^* / v$, $j = 1, 2$,
- $\mathbb{V}(S_j^*) = \sigma^2 \cdot v_j^* (v - v_j^*) / (v - 1) = V(v^*)$, $j = 1, 2$,

where V is a positive function, and $v = v_1 + v_2$, $S = S_1 + S_2$ and $\sigma^2 = \sum_{ji} (Y_{ji} - S/v)^2 \cdot O_{ji} / v$ are permutationally invariant nonnull quantities. Thus, for any given pair of positive permutation actual sample sizes (v_1^*, v_2^*), the two permutation sampling totals S_1^* and S_2^* have the same variance and their correlation coefficient is $\rho(S_1^*, S_2^*) = -1$, because their sum S is a permutation invariant quantity. Hence, we may write:

- $\mathbb{E}[T^*(a^*, b^*)] = a^* \cdot S \cdot v_1^* - b^* \cdot S \cdot v_2^* = 0$,
- $\mathbb{V}[T^*(a^*, b^*)] = a^{*2} V(v^*) + 2a^* b^* V(v^*) + b^{*2} V(v^*) = (a^* + b^*)^2 V(v^*)$.

The solutions to these equations are $a^* = (v_2^* / v_1^*)^{1/2}$ and $b^* = (v_1^* / v_2^*)^{1/2}$, ignoring an inessential positive coefficient.

Hence, for $C = 2$ and $V = 1$, the test statistic, the sub-distributions of which are approximately invariant with respect to permutation of actual sample sizes of valid data because they are permutationally invariant in mean value and variance, takes the form

$$T^* = S_1^* \cdot (v_2^* / v_1^*)^{1/2} - S_2^* \cdot (v_1^* / v_2^*)^{1/2}.$$

If there are no missing values, so that $v_j^* = n_j$, $j = 1, 2$, the latter test is permutationally equivalent to the standard two-sample permutation test for comparison of locations $T^* \approx \sum_i Y_{1i}^*$.

In the case of $C > 2$ and again with $V = 1$, one approximate solution is

$$T_C^* = \sum_{j=1}^{c} \{ S_j^* \cdot (v - v_j^*) / v_j^{*1/2} - (S - S_j^*) \cdot v_j^* / (v - v_j^*)^{1/2} \}^2.$$

This test statistic may be seen as a direct combination of C partial dependent tests, each obtained by a permutation comparison of the jth group with respect to all other $C - 1$ groups pooled together. Also, in the case of complete data, when there are no missing values, this test is equivalent to the permutation test for a standard one-way ANOVA layout, provided that sample sizes are balanced, $n_j = m$, $j = 1, \ldots, C$, whereas in the unbalanced cases the two solutions, although not coincident, are very close to each other.

One more solution may be obtained by the direct NPC of all pairwise comparisons:

$$T_{2C}^* = \Sigma_{r<j}(T_{rj}^*)^2,$$

where $T_{rj}^* = S_r^* \cdot (v_j^* / v_r^*)^{1/2} - S_j^* \cdot (v_r^* / v_j^*)^{1/2}, \ 1 \le r < j \le C$.

Of course, if $V > 1$, a non-parametric combination will result. Hence, to test $H_0 : \{\cap_h H_{0h}^{\mathbf{Y|O}}\}$ against $H_1 : \{\cap_h H_{1h}^{\mathbf{Y|O}}\}$, the solution becomes $T'' = \psi(\lambda_1, ..., \lambda_V)$, where ψ is any member of the class C, and λ_h is the partial p-value of either

$$T_{Ch}^* = \sum_{j=1}^{c} \left\{ S_{hj}^* \cdot \left(\frac{v_h - v_{hj}^*}{v_{hj}^*} \right)^{1/2} - (S_h - S_{hj}^*) \cdot \left(\frac{v_{hj}^*}{v_h - v_{hj}^*} \right)^{1/2} \right\}^2,$$

or

$$T_{2Ch}^* = \Sigma_{r<j} \left(S_{hr}^* \cdot (v_{hj}^* / v_{hr}^*)^{1/2} - S_{hj}^* \cdot (v_{hr}^* / v_{hj}^*)^{1/2} \right)^2,$$

each relative to the hth component variable, $h = 1, ..., V$.

For MNAR models, again in a nonparametric way, we must also combine the V test statistics on the components of the inclusion indicator $\mathbf{O}$, provided that all partial tests are marginally unbiased (see Sect. 4.2.1). More specifically, to test $H_0 : \{\cap_h H_{0h}^{\mathbf{O}} \cap \cap_h H_{0h}^{\mathbf{Y|O}}\}$ against $H_1 : \{\cup_h H_{1h}^{\mathbf{O}} \cup \cup_h H_{1h}^{\mathbf{Y|O}}\}$ we must now combine V tests $T_h^{*\mathbf{O}}$ and V tests $T_h^{*\mathbf{Y|O}}$, $h = 1, ..., V$. Hence (with obvious notation)

$$T'' = \psi(\lambda_1^{\mathbf{O}}, ..., \lambda_V^{\mathbf{O}}; \lambda_1^{\mathbf{Y|O}}, ..., \lambda_V^{\mathbf{Y|O}}).$$

For each of the V subhypotheses $H_{0h}^{\mathbf{O}}$ against $H_{1h}^{\mathbf{O}}$, a permutation statistic such as Pearson's chi-square or any other suitable test statistic for proper testing of categorical data may be used (for instance, when $C=2$ and restricted alternatives are of interest, Fisher's exact probability test may be appropriate). This combined permutation test has good general asymptotic properties. In particular, under very mild conditions, if best univariate partial tests are used, then the combined test is asymptotically best in the same sense.

5.5   Botulinum Data

In this section, we consider a real case study, related to a preliminary double-blind, placebo controlled, randomized clinical trial with a 6-month follow-up period. The purpose of this trial is to evaluate the effectiveness of type A botulinum toxin to treat myofascial pain symptoms and to reduce muscle hyperactivity in bruxers. In order to do this, 20 patients (10 males, 10 females; aged between 25 and 45) with clinical diagnosis of bruxism and with myofascial pain of masticatory muscles were enrolled.These patients were randomly divided into two groups of 10 patients. A group received botulinum toxin injections—BTX-A (treated group) and the other group was treated with saline placebo injections (control group). Several clinical variables (in the medical literature, same as "end-points") were assessed at baseline time, at 1 week, 1 month, and 6-month follow-up appointments, along with electromyography (EMG) recordings of muscle activity in different conditions. Clinical end points are as follows:

- *pain at rest* (DR), *at phoning* (DF), and *at chewing* (DM), assessed by means of a visual analog scale (VAS) from 0 to 10, with the extremes being "no pain" and "pain as bad as the patient has ever experienced" respectively;
- *mastication efficiency* (CM), assessed by a VAS from 0 to 10, the extremes of which were "eating only semiliquid" and "eating solid hard food";
- *maximum nonassisted* (Mas) and *assisted* (Maf) mouth opening (in millimeters), *protrusive* (Mp), and *laterotrusive left* (Mll) and *right* (Mlr) movements (in millimeters);
- *functional limitation* (LF) during usual jaw movements (0, absent; 1, slight; 2, moderate; 3, intense; 4, severe);

At the same time as the clinical evaluations, all patients underwent EMG recordings of left and right anterior and posterior temporalis muscles at rest (LTA, RTA, LTP, RTP, respectively) and left and right masseter muscles at rest (LMM, RMM); left and right anterior temporalis muscles during maximum voluntary clenching (LTA11, RTA11) and during clenching on cotton rolls (LTA11c, RTA11c); masseter muscles during maximum voluntary clenching (LMM11, RMM11) and during clenching on cotton rolls (LMM11c, RMM11c).

1. Hence, we are in presence of a multivariate problem whit repeated measures and missing data. In particular, for each of $n=20$ $(n_1 = n_2 = 10)$ units in $C=2$ experimental situations (which represent the two levels of the treatment), a V-dimensional non-degenerate variable ($V=24$) is observed on $k=4$ different time occasions. Note that in this longitudinal study the number of observed variables in different time points is much higher than the number of subjects ($V \cdot k \gg n$), thus parametric tests are not available. Furthermore, since all variables may be informative for differentiating two groups, the NPC approach properly applies when analyzing these data. Classic parametric tests or even rank tests in such situations may fail to take into account the dependence structure across variables and time points.

The whole data set is denoted by:

$$\mathbf{X} = \{X_{hji}(t), t = 1,\ldots,k, i = 1,\ldots,n_j, j = 1,2, h = 1,\ldots,V\}$$
$$= \{\mathbf{X}_{hji}, i = 1,\ldots,n_j, j = 1,2, h = 1,\ldots,V\},$$

where $\mathbf{X}_{hji} = \{X_{hji}(t), t = 1,\ldots,k\}$.

In order to take account of different baseline observations, assumed to have the role of covariates, the $k-1$ V-dimensional differences $D_{hji}(t) = X_{hji}(1) - X_{hji}(t)$,

$t = 2,\ldots,k,\ \ i = 1,\ldots,n_j,\ \ j = 1,2,\ \ h = 1,\ldots,: V$, are considered in the analysis. Hence the hypothesis testing problem related to the hth variable may be formalized as

$$H_{0h} : \left\{ \bigcap_{t=2}^{k} \left[D_{h1}(t) \overset{d}{=} D_{h2}(t) \right] \right\} = \left\{ \bigcap_{t=2}^{k} H_{0ht} \right\}, h = 1,\ldots,V,$$

against the alternative:

$$H_{1h} : \left\{ \bigcup_{t=2}^{k} H_{1ht} \right\}, h = 1,\ldots,V,$$

where $H_{1ht} : D_{h1}(t) \overset{d}{>} D_{h2}(t)$ or $D_{h1}(t) \overset{d}{<} D_{h2}(t)$ according to which kind of stochastic dominance is of interest for the hth variable. The alternative hypothesis is that patients treated with the botulinum toxin had lower values than those treated with the placebo (i.e., differences between baseline values and follow-up values tend to increase, for which the $\overset{d}{>}$ dominance is appropriate), except for variables: ME, Mas, Maf, Mp, Mll, Mlr, E, and T, where the placebo group is expected to have lower values than the toxin group, for which the $\overset{d}{<}$ is then appropriate.

References

Agresti A. Categorical data analysis. Hoboken: Wiley; 2002.

Blair RC, Higgins JJ, Karniski W, Kromrey JD. A study of multivariate permutation tests which may replace Hotelling's t^2 test in prescribed circumstances. Multivar Behav Res. 1994;29:141–63.

Chung JH, Fraser DAS. Randomization tests for a multivariate two-sample problem. J Am Stat Assoc. 1958;53:729–35.

Cressie NAC, Read TRC. Goodness of fit statistics for discrete multivariate data. New York: Springer; 1988.

Crowder MJ, Hand DJ. Analysis of repeated measures. London: Chapman & Hall; 1990.

Diggle PJ, Liang KY, Zeger SL. Analysis of longitudinal data. Oxford: Oxford University Press; 2002.

Dempster AP, Laird NM, Rubin DB. Maximum likelihood from incomplete data via the EM algorithm. J R Stat Soc B. 1977;39:1–38.

Lehmann EL. Parametric versus nonparametrics: two alternative methodologies. J Nonparametr Stat. 2009;21:397–405.

Little RJA, Rubin DB. Statistical analysis with missing data. New York: Wiley; 1987.

Pesarin F, Salmaso L. Permutation tests for complex data: theory, applications and software. Chichester: Wiley; 2010.